J. Madison Watson

Watson's Manual of Calisthenics

A Systematic Drill-Book without Apparatus

J. Madison Watson

Watson's Manual of Calisthenics
A Systematic Drill-Book without Apparatus

ISBN/EAN: 9783744736701

Printed in Europe, USA, Canada, Australia, Japan

Cover: Foto ©Paul-Georg Meister /pixelio.de

More available books at **www.hansebooks.com**

WATSON'S

MANUAL OF CALISTHENICS:

A SYSTEMATIC DRILL-BOOK

WITHOUT APPARATUS, FOR

SCHOOLS, FAMILIES, AND GYMNASIUMS.

WITH

MUSIC TO ACCOMPANY THE EXERCISES.

Illustrated from Original Designs.

By J. MADISON WATSON.

CHICAGO:
GEO. & C. W. SHERWOOD, 118 LAKE STREET.
NEW YORK AND PHILADELPHIA:
SCHERMERHORN, BANCROFT & CO.
1864.

Entered according to Act of Congress, in the year one thousand eight hundred and sixty-four,

BY J. MADISON WATSON,

In the Clerk's Office of the District Court of the United States for the Southern District of New York.

RENNIE, SHEA & LINDSAY,
STEREOTYPERS AND ELECTROTYPERS,
81, 83, & 85 CENTRE-STREET,
NEW YORK.

PRINTED BY
C. A. ALVORD,
15 Vandewater-st.,
NEW YORK.

PREFACE.

ALTHOUGH this treatise is taken almost wholly from "WATSON'S HAND-BOOK OF CALISTHENICS AND GYMNASTICS," such changes and additions have been made as render it complete in itself. Its object is to serve as a Manual of Calisthenics for individuals and families, and a systematic Drill-Book for schools and gymnasiums, affording the most extended and varied course of physical exercises, without the aid of apparatus, ever published.

The INTRODUCTION embraces all needful directions, rules, and explanations for instructors and students, and full and satisfactory sections on Phonetics and Respiration.

The second division, CALISTHENICS, will enable teachers to give physical training its due prominence in primary instruction, and afford students of all grades, in connection with the many excellent works now published on mental and moral training, the necessary additional facilities for the acquisition of a symmetrical education, with its attendant blessings. The *elementary* movements are sufficiently numerous and varied to secure the requisite simultaneous activity of the mental and physical powers, and call into play all of the joints, sinews, and muscles. After they are mastered, the more beautiful and effective *combined* movements may be executed without previous practice, simply by employing appropriate words of command.

All varieties of marking time while executing the movements are given, including counting, Phonetics, Recitations, and Music. Nineteen pieces of appropriate *Piano-forte Music* are introduced in their proper connections. Those not composed expressly for this work are selected and arranged from the choicest productions of the ablest masters.

To G. F. Bristow and H. B. Dodworth, gentlemen whose merits as musicians and composers are generally recognized, the author is greatly indebted for valuable assistance, freely and generously afforded, in this department of his work. He is also happy to acknowledge himself under equal obligations to Miss C. Hutchings, of New York, for corresponding aid.

All the exercises are arranged in accordance with well-known principles of Anatomy, Physiology, and Hygiene. They have been thoroughly and repeatedly tested in gymnasiums and schools, invariably securing the happiest results. They are especially valuable in cases of incipient consumption, dyspepsia, and general muscular weakness, insuring the regulation of associated, and the equal development of antagonistic groups of muscles.

In order to present successfully a *new system* of Calisthenics, a series of ILLUSTRATIONS from *original designs* is indispensable. The CUTS that accompany these exercises were prepared expressly for this work, illustrating positions actually taken and movements executed by the author. They were drawn on wood by Geo. G. White and E. Vedder, and engraved by N. Orr & Co.

Practiced habitually and energetically in youth, the author believes that the following exercises can not fail to give the student grace, agility, suppleness, a good eye, and a ready hand,—as well as robust health, solid strength, and power of endurance.

New York, *June*, 1864.

CONTENTS.

I. INTRODUCTION

Instruction of Assistants	9
Commands	10
Position of the Students	10
Time and Rhythmus	12
Vocal Exercises with Calisthenics	14
Music with Calisthenics	14
Formation of the Class	15
Instruction of the Class	18
Instruction of the School	19
Calisthenic Hall	20
Costume	22
General Divisions	25
Oral Elements	26
Respiration	27

II. GENERAL EXERCISES.

CALISTHENICS	31
CHEST EXERCISE	32
First Series	32
Second Series	36
Third Series	36
Fourth Series	37
VOCAL EXERCISES	39
Counting	39
Phonetics	40
Recitations	41
Vocal Music	42
Instrumental Music	43
Music for Chest Exercise	46
SHOULDER EXERCISE	50
First Series	50
Second Series	53
Music for Shoulder Exercise	48
ELBOW EXERCISE	59
First Series	59

CONTENTS.

  Second Series 64
  Music for Elbow Exercise 54
ARM AND HAND EXERCISE 65
  First Series 65
  Second Series 69
  Third Series 73
  Fourth Series 76
  Fifth Series 79
  Music for Arm and Hand Exercise 56
HEAD AND NECK EXERCISE 87
  First Series 87
  Second Series 89
  Music for Head and Neck Exercise 83
TRUNK AND WAIST EXERCISE 90
  First Series 90
  Second Series 93
  Music for Trunk and Waist Exercise 84
KNEE EXERCISE 95
  First Series 95
  Second Series 99
  Music for Knee Exercise 85
LEG AND FOOT EXERCISE 106
  First Series 106
  Second Series 108
  Third Series 113
  Fourth Series 117
  Fifth Series 120
  Sixth Series 123
  Seventh Series 126
  Music for Leg and Foot Exercise 102
COMBINED EXERCISES 130
  First Series 130
  Second Series 134
  Third Series 135
  Fourth Series 139
  Fifth Series 140

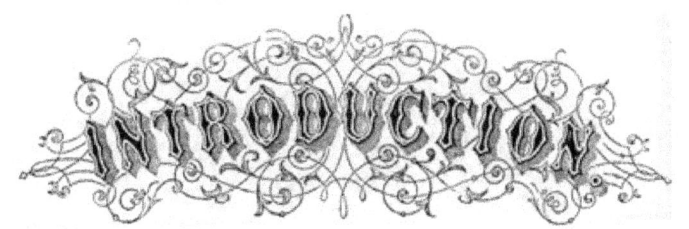

INTRODUCTION.

CALISTHEN'ICS, from the two Greek words KALOS, signifying *beautiful*, and STHENOS, *strength*, is the name applied in this work to an extended course of exercises, *performed without the aid of technical apparatus*, which is designed to further the proportionate development of the body; render the joints more flexible in all directions; give the pleasing and graceful appearance of firmness, steadiness, and dexterity in the positions and in the use of the limbs; and secure physical beauty, muscular strength, and robust health.

INSTRUCTION OF ASSISTANTS.

IN Calisthenics, as in all other things taught, every principal is responsible for the instruction of his school. He should assemble his assistants or monitors together for theoretical and practical instruction as often as he may judge necessary. When he is unable to attend to this duty in person, it may be discharged by the vice-principal, or an instructor specially appointed for the purpose.

When instruction is given to assistants, or a number of teachers, they should be required to explain the positions and movements of the different classes of exercise, and to put them into practical operation. Each command in a lesson, at the theoretical instruction, should be given by the principal, and then repeated in succession by his assistants, so that while they become **habituated** to the commands, uniformity **may be** established in the manner of giving them.

COMMANDS.

THERE are three kinds: the command of *caution*, or attention; the *preparatory command*, which indicates the position that is to be taken, or the class of movements that is to be executed; and the command of *execution*, or the part of the command which causes an execution.

The tone of command should be animated, distinct, and of a loudness proportioned to the size of the room and the number of students under instruction.

The commands of caution and the preparatory commands are herein distinguished by *italics;* those of execution, by CAPITALS. The preparatory commands are given distinctly, with an ascending progression in the tone of command, but always in such a manner that the tone of execution may be more energetic and elevated. The divisions are indicated by a dash. The parts of commands which are placed in a parenthesis are not pronounced. Commands in music, on page 43.

POSITION OF THE STUDENT.

THE position of the student, when not otherwise directed, will always be the *military* or *fundamental position*, as shown in the accompanying figures. At the command, ATTENTION, or POSITION,

1. HEELS TOGETHER. The heels are placed on the same line, as near each other as the conformation of the student will permit.

2. FEET OUTWARD. The feet are turned out equally, forming with each other something less than a right angle.

3. KNEES JOINED. The knees are joined and kept straight, without stiffness.

POSITION OF THE STUDENT.   11

4. BODY ERECT. The body is erect on the hips, inclining a little forward.

5. SHOULDERS BACK. Both shoulders form a straight line, at right angles with the neck and head, and fall equally.

6. ARMS DOWN. The arms hang naturally.

7. ELBOWS IN. The elbows are held near the body, but not hugged to the sides.

8. HANDS OUTWARD. The palms of the hands are turned a little to the front, and the little fingers touch the outsides of the thigh.

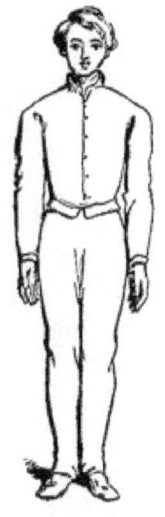
FIG. 5.

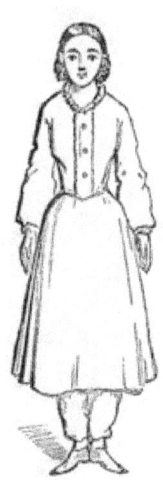
FIG. 6.

9. HEAD UP. The head is held erect and square to the front, without constraint.

10. EYES FRONT. The eyes are fixed on some object in front of the body, about twenty feet forward on the ground, when not directed to the instructor.

11. MOUTH SHUT. *The breathing should in all cases be carried on through the nose.*

COMMENCING POSITION. The position in which the body is when about to execute a certain movement, or class of movements, is called the commencing position of that movement. This position may therefore vary almost infinitely.

POSITIONS TAKEN. The positions commanded to be taken refer always to that part of the body last mentioned as under command; and when taken, they must be kept until others are commanded. When two, three, or more parts of the body are included in the command, their position should be taken together.

TIME AND RHYTHMUS.

IN order that Calisthenics may produce the most desirable effects on the mental and spiritual nature of man, as well as on his physical, it is not only necessary that the movements have a determined form and order of execution, but that they have a determined *time*, the rhythmus or division of which is well established in the mind.

The measure of time must also be viewed in a special way, as far as it regards Calisthenics. If we see a whole series of movements, either one exercise repeatedly executed according to a certain law, or different exercises following each other according to a similar law, then we have the rhythmus; the movements become rhythmical, and the various motions appear as parts of a certain measure of time. Military marching may serve as an instance: it consists of one principal movement, the repeatedly executed pace, which, being alternately done by both feet, appears as a double movement, which in its repetitions produces the movement of walking; and this, if the same time is observed for both feet and for the repetitions, becomes a rhythmical walking or marching. Each pace is a part of a measure which finishes with the setting down of the advanced foot.

The special rhythmical relations of walking and marching, as well as in general of all the advancing foot movements, are made sensible either by directing our attention principally to one foot while the other is comparatively disregarded, and thereby to our imagination the steps of the first foot appear the heavier and stronger; or the rhythmus may be observed by marking more prominently the steps of one of the feet, or in general certain steps, which are, so to speak, somewhat more accentuated, either by a really more vigorous tread, or by resting longer with one foot on the ground, or by executing at certain steps corresponding movements of other limbs (clapping together of the hands, for instance, inclination of the upper part of the body, etc.): in this way originate rhythmical forms of time, which show themselves as determined metrical articulations.

As each simple movement involves a certain measure of time, so the compound movements, and those which follow each other, must be executed in a certain measure of time or in so many single consecutive measures. It is an indispensable quality of the rational instructor to divide each class of movements into its constituent motions or elements, and to mark them during their performance by counting. In this way the student becomes conscious of the form and signification of each class of movements, and the exercises become *conscious actions*. This is also a reason why Calisthenics are not only a means for the development of the body, but also for that of the mental and spiritual man. The mind is taught to govern the body, and every articulation and limb is habituated to a prompt and ready obedience to the will.

Calisthenic exercises have their greatest value when done by many together, and under the direction of an experienced instructor. Then an orderly and exact execution of the movements is only rendered possible by a perfect rhythmus, which is made evident to the eye or ear of each member of the class. As a majority of English songs, and nearly all marches, dances, and other pieces of music that are employed to secure simultaneous movements, are in *eights*, the rhythmus should be octosyllabic. The most *useful* mode of securing concert is by employing the voice; the most *pleasing*, instrumental music.

VOCAL EXERCISES WITH CALISTHENICS.

BE the instrumental music never so good, the instructor should always conduct a portion of the movements to vocal exercises.

1. COUNTING. Let the members of the class count continuously in concert, from one to eight inclusive, at an average rate of ninety in a minute, which rate may be most readily determined by the use of a metronome. The instructor gives the words of command, and the students take the required positions and execute all the movements in exact time as marked by the counting. For Varieties, see No. 28, page 39.

2. PHONETICS. When phonetics are employed, all the members of the division will produce the tonics consecutively, as arranged in the Table of Oral Elements, p. 26, uttering each one eight times, or adopt some other variety of No. 29, page 40. Combinations formed by prefixing and affixing subtonics and atonics to the tonics will be employed in like manner.

3. RECITATIONS AND SONGS. Spirited recitations in octosyllabic verse—narrative, descriptive, and lyric; national odes, and battle-pieces, should frequently be used with Calisthenics to mark the time. Appropriate selections are given in text-books. Let the pieces be so recited that the poetry may address itself to the heart; that the tones of the voice may be more akin to music than ordinary speech; that the prosody may be carefully observed, giving every line its proper part in the melody, without spoiling the sense by a sing-song cadence. Vocal music should also be employed in this connection.

MUSIC WITH CALISTHENICS.

IN order to awaken a lively and abiding interest in calisthenic and gymnastic exercises, and to secure an enthusiasm and a fascination that shall convert indolence and sluggishness into cheerful and vigorous activity, it will be found absolutely necessary to employ instrumental music.

The best music for this purpose is furnished by a brass band; and is specially appropriate for public inspection or exhibition. There are many single instruments that are easily obtained. A drum, a tambourine, a triangle, or even a common plow-clevis, while less pleasing than some other instruments, secures most perfect concert. The flute, the guitar, and the violin are excellent; but the piano, all things considered, is preferable. Appropriate music, specially arranged for the last-named instrument, is introduced in the body of this work. For commands, and further explanations, see p. 43.

FORMATION OF THE CLASS.

TO execute the classes of movements well from the different positions, the students must be placed in a definite order, and this is called the *formation of the class.* The

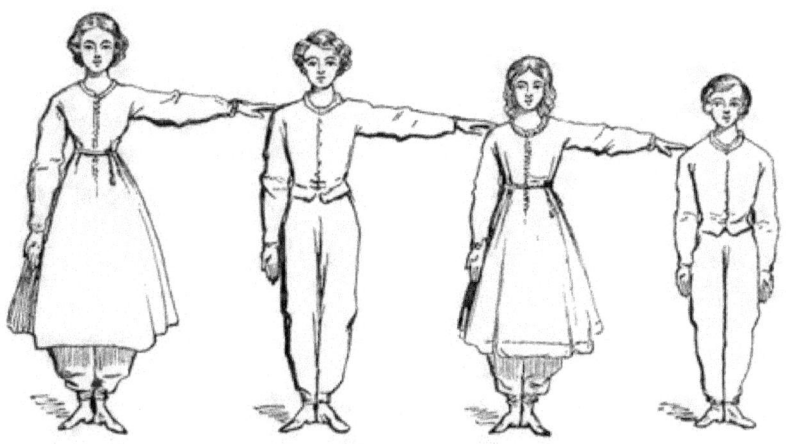

Fig. 7.

formation depends on the *kind* of exercise, and also the *place* of exercise. When the space permits, all the students are to be placed abreast.

When the students have assembled, or the hour for the exercise has arrived, the order is, *Class*—FALL IN; on which the students place themselves in front of the instructor according to their height, beside each other in one rank, so near as to *slightly* touch each other with their elbows, and yet leaving room enough for their arms to swing. The tallest student stands at the left of the instructor, and the shortest at his right. In most exercises each student must have sufficient space to move his limbs in all directions without being hindered; for this purpose the open formation is chosen, which is made from the close formation at the order, *Take your Distance*—MARCH!

At the announcing order, each student, except the last, lays his left hand on his left neighbor's right shoulder; and at the command, MARCH! the student at the instructor's right remains in his place, while every other one moves away from his neighbor at his left, until his own left arm and hand are freely stretched out, so that the points of his fingers only touch his neighbor's right shoulder, as in Fig. 7.

At the command, POSITION! the stretched arms are simultaneously placed down by the side, and the students take the *fundamental* or *military position*.

If the room will not admit of one expanded line, two or three may be formed in like manner; however, at the least, from four to five feet apart from each other. The first student in the second line at the instructor's right will be the next taller than the last student of the front line at the instructor's left. When facing toward the instructor, the students of the back lines will *cover square*—that is, stand *exactly* behind the ones in front.

For some movements, the open formation just described does not give a sufficient distance. In such cases, at the order, *Take a double distance*—MARCH! wider distance is taken, by each student placing himself so far from his neighbors, that he can with his stretched arms and fingers touch the tips of the fingers of the stretched arms of his neighbors. This formation, however, requires a greater longitudinal space, and makes it more difficult, if there is a great number of students, to overlook them.

FORMATION OF THE CLASS. 17

In such cases, when the students are in the position illustrated by Fig. 7, the instructor will first command : *In line (or each line)*—COUNT TWOS ; and the students count from right to left, commencing with the shortest one in the rank nearest the instructor, pronouncing distinctly, in the same tone, without hurry and without turning the head, *one, two; one, two,* &c., according to the place each one occupies.

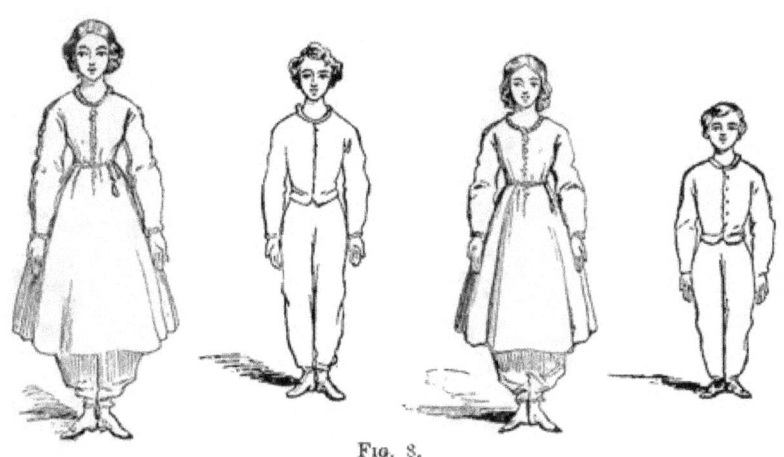

FIG. 8.

Now follows the command, *Twos, one pace forward*—MARCH! on which the *ones* retain their places, and the *twos* take a step forward of about thirty inches, and join heels, as seen in Fig. 8. In this formation, longitudinal space is saved, and supervision made easy. The distances that now result must be strictly retained, as they are the most convenient to enable each student to take all the positions of the body, without inconvenience to his neighbors.

As soon as the necessary formation is executed, each individual must assume the *fundamental* or *military position*. From this position all others proceed, and also many of the movements. If, at the order of the instructor, any other commencing position has been assumed, and we wish that the fundamental position shall be taken, it is done at the command, ATTENTION! or, POSITION!

INSTRUCTION OF THE CLASS.

IN class drill, or in a small school where but one teacher is employed, the object being the instruction and improvement of the students, the instructor never requires a position to be taken, or a movement to be executed, until he has given an exact explanation of it; and he executes, himself, the movement which he commands, so as to join example to precept. He accustoms the students to take, by themselves, the exact position which is explained; and sees that all the movements are performed without precipitation.

Each movement should be understood before passing to another. After the movements have been properly executed in the order laid down in a general division, the instructor no longer confines himself to that order; but, on the contrary, he should vary the exercises frequently, that he may elicit thought, judge of the intelligence of the students, and call into action, alternately, various sets of muscles.

The instructor allows the students to rest at the end of each part of the lessons, and oftener, if he thinks proper, especially at the commencement; for this purpose he commands—Rest.

At this command, the student is no longer required to preserve immobility. He may change his position, but may not leave the ranks. If the instructor wishes merely to relieve the attention of the student, he commands, *Right foot in place*—Rest; the student is then not required to preserve his immobility, but he always keeps the foot named in the preparatory command on the line, and carries the other foot six inches to the rear, slightly bending the advanced knee, and lets the weight of the body fall mainly on the foot in the rear.

When the instructor wishes to commence the instruction, he commands, *Attention*—Class; when the students take their position, remain motionless, and fix their attention.

During the initial exercises, and until the student has acquired the ability to execute readily the classes of movements of the positions under consideration at the time, all the students will *count* as described on pp. 14 and 39.

At the commencement, slow movements should be practiced, then quicker ones; afterward the command for rapid and slow movements should be given so as to take the pupil by surprise, and the same with regard to one member only, or several together.

Exercises should always be commenced as well as finished gently. This is especially important for beginners, as they are sometimes injured, and their progress retarded, by too severe efforts at first.

The instructor will remember, that the organs or parts are to be developed and strengthened by moderate and prolonged exertions, rather than by violent and fitful ones. The weaker organs or limbs should always receive more attention, and be more frequently subjected to exercises specially adapted to their invigoration.

All violent exertions should be made when the stomach is empty, or nearly so. The best times for the more active calisthenic exercises are early in the morning, and toward evening; when practiced at school, the best times are the middle of the forenoon, and toward the close of the afternoon session. They should not be practiced immediately after meals, nor very near the time for eating, as digestion is never well performed when the system is in an agitated or exhausted condition.

INSTRUCTION OF THE SCHOOL.

THE harmony so indispensable in the movements of the several classes of a large school, or of two or more schools, can only be attained by the use of the same commands, the same principles, and the same mode of execution. Hence, in order to render general exercises most interesting, effective, and useful, all instructors will conform themselves, without addition or curtailment, to what will herein be prescribed, until a perfect mastery is secured.

The movements, as described from the different positions named in this work, are intended for separate classes, or schools where there is sufficient space for students to stand in lines far enough apart to prevent their hands or feet coming in contact. The intelligent instructor will not find it difficult, however, to make such modifications and omissions as will enable him to conduct exercises successfully when the students are seated, or when they are standing in a compact body.

In the chapel, or other room for school drill, the students will have seats assigned solely with reference to their height: those that are shortest will be seated nearest the principal's platform.

The exercises of each lesson will be executed several times in the order in which they are arranged, and the lessons will be introduced consecutively; but as soon as the school shall be confirmed in the principles of Calisthenics, and taught to perform all the exercises with the utmost precision, the order of the positions, of the movements, and of the general divisions, may be varied.

During a *public* inspection or exhibition, the instructor will employ only the commands necessary to vary the usual order of exercises. An occasional departure from this rule may be advisable, to impart greater animation. He will not execute, himself, the movements he commands; but he may indicate by gesture both the nature and the direction of the movements. To insure promptitude and perfect uniformity, an assistant, or an intelligent student, occupying a position in front, may execute the movements simultaneously with the school.

CALISTHENIC HALL.

THE floor of a calisthenic hall should be streaked or inlaid, as shown in Fig. 9. The lines must be about *thirty* inches apart, both lengthwise and crosswise of the room. Each intersection forms a standing. Many classes of exercise may be executed when all the standings are occupied; but in that event it will be found necessary to make some modifications and omissions.

The preferable mode is, after the instructor has sized the ranks, to form the whole school into two equal divisions—

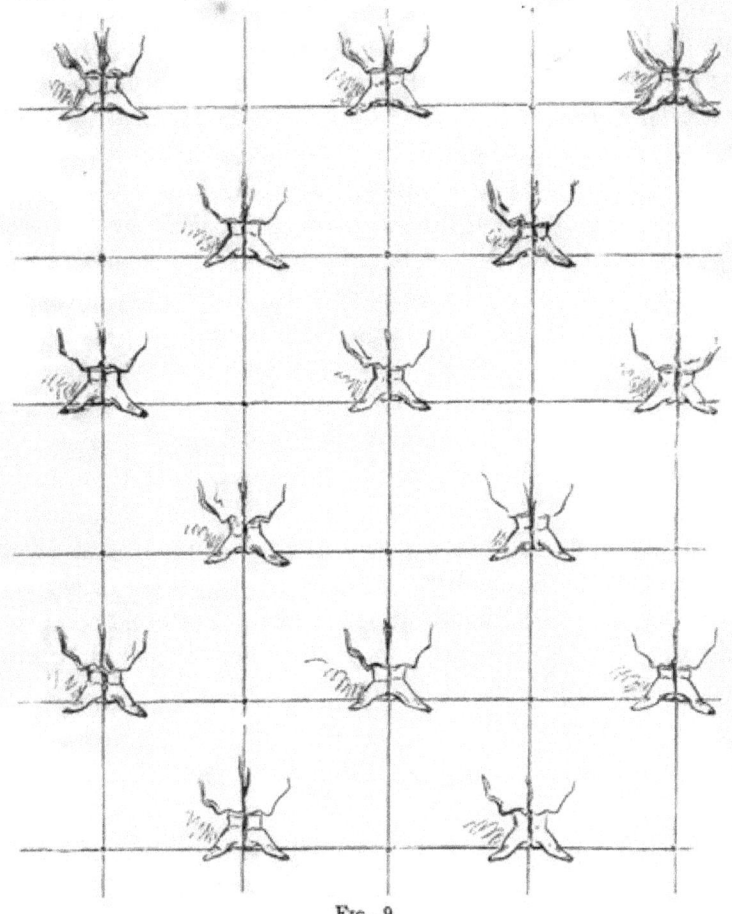

Fig. 9.

all the odd lines, from side to side, constituting the first division; and the even lines, the second. Then one division will rest while the other is under drill; or they will occupy the hall on alternate days, or during different hours of the same day.

The formation of the division under drill will be as follows: At the command, *First (or second) division*—FALL IN, every member of the division (knowing his own relative height, rank, and position) will at once take his standing. The shortest student in the division will occupy the first standing at the teacher's right, in the front rank; and the tallest one, the last standing at the teacher's left, in the rank furthest back. The ranks will occupy every second line, commencing with the second one front.

As soon as this formation is secured, the instructor commands, *In every rank*—COUNT TWOS; and the students count *twos*, as directed on page 17. At the command, *Twos, one standing forward*—MARCH, the *twos* step forward (*left foot first*) and occupy the standings immediately in front, thus completing the formation as represented by the feet in Fig. 9.

At the conclusion of the exercise, or preparatory to marching, the instructor commands, *Twos, one standing backward*—MARCH; and the *twos* step backward (*left foot first*) and occupy their original standings in the ranks.

The temperature of a calisthenic hall should be kept at from 63 to 70 degrees; but during the continuance of the exercises the windows should be opened, so that the room may be thoroughly ventilated. All heavy and unnecessary clothing should be removed. At the close of the exercise, when the quick movements and changing evolutions of the limbs and the joints have increased the animal heat and produced a sensible perspiration, the windows must be closed, and all draughts of air avoided. A perfect ventilation, however, must be secured at all times.

COSTUME.

IN arranging a costume[1] for calisthenic and gymnastic exercises, we must take into account what may be regarded as the elementary requisites of all dress: that it be

---

[1] **Costume.**—The author, in the preparation of this article, has incorporated valuable ideas from an able paper in the Atlantic Monthly, entitled *Daily Beauty*. A perusal of that paper is earnestly recommended.

comfortable and decent, convenient and suitable, beautiful in form and color, simple, genuine, harmonious with Nature and itself.

The first two requisites of dress are easily attained; for only a sufficiency of suitable covering is necessary to them. Dress, however, should not only secure these points, but *seem* to secure them; for, as to others than the wearer, what is the difference between sweltering and seeming to swelter, shivering and seeming to shiver?

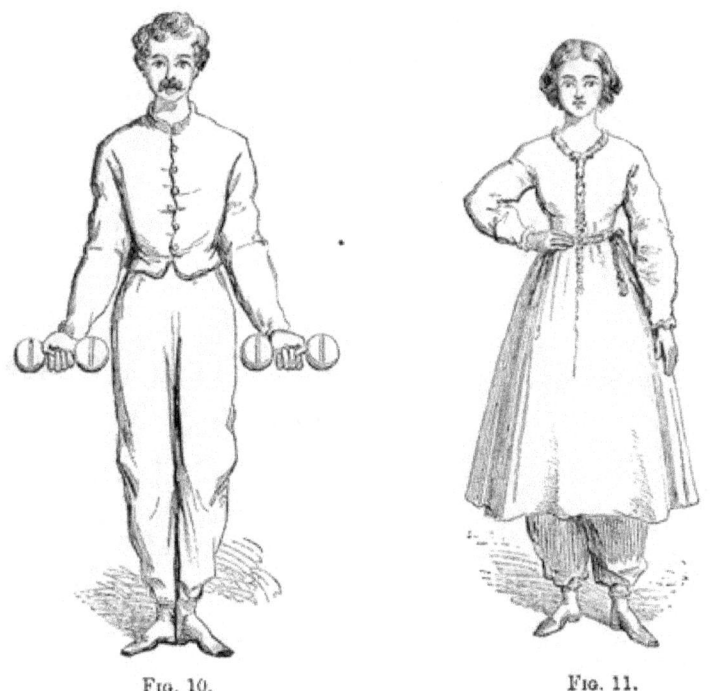

Fig. 10. Fig. 11.

Convenience, which is to be distinguished from mere bodily comfort, is the next essential of becoming dress. A man should not wear a Spanish cloak while using a flail or a pair of Indian clubs; a woman should not make butter in large hanging-sleeves, nor walk on muddy roads in long, trailing skirts. No beauty of form or splendor of material in costume can compensate for manifest inconvenience to the wearer. No dress is sanctioned by good taste which does not permit, and seem to permit, the easy performance of any movement proper to the wearer's age and condition in life; for it defies the very first law of the mixed arts—*fitness*.

Form is the most important element of the absolute beauty of dress, as it is of all arts that appeal to the eye. The lines of costume should, in every part, conform to those of nature, or be in harmony with them. In color, another important element of beauty, no fine effects of costume are to be attained without broad masses of pure and positive tints. The various tints of brown may be employed with fine effect in composing a costume; but the best hues for a calisthenic dress are blue, gray, red, green, purple, and scarlet.

The illustrations here introduced give a correct idea of the style of the costume best adapted to calisthenic and gymnastic exercises. Indeed, all the elementary requisites of dress are here combined, rendering its adaptation perfect to every purpose for which a costume is intended.

In Fig. 11, the drapery is not, as is too frequently the case, deformed and hateful; for its lines conform to those of the parts of the person which it conceals. With what completeness, ease, and comfort it clothes the entire figure of the wearer! There is not a line about it which indicates compression, or one expressive of heedless laxity. Both limbs and trunk are amply draped; and yet how plainly it is seen that the wearer is well developed and untortured. The waist, girdled in at the proper place, is of its natural size. How expressive the figure is of health, and grace, and bounteous fullness of life!

The dress opens in front, and is both more convenient and more beautiful than one which opens behind. It is so constructed that the wearer's limbs are as free as air; that she can even clap her hands, with arms vertical, above her head without the slightest discomfort. The gown is short, and the skirt is full, reaching only to about the middle of the calf of the leg; and therefore, though worn without hoops, it does not fall closely around the figure. The trowsers, which are also full, are gathered in at the ankle by a plain band, which has a small ruffle at the lower edge. The trimming, in moderate quantity, is put on the principal seams and the edges. The material, at all seasons of the year, both for male and female, should be flannel.

It will be observed that the gentleman's dress (Fig. 10) is loose and comfortable. The primary object of the costume is not to exhibit rounded and shapely limbs and well-developed muscles, but to give ease and comfort to the student in all of his positions and movements. The military jacket, without unnecessary padding, is selected. It has no useless skirt, and the collar is neither high nor stiff. The trowsers, which are very loose, are gathered in and buttoned at the ankle, or fastened with an elastic band or a small strap.

Students may exercise in their street dresses. The gentlemen will remove their coats. The ladies will use elastic bands to sustain their skirts, so that the wearer's legs and feet may have free play. Bathing dresses will very generally be found pretty and appropriate for these exercises.

GENERAL DIVISIONS.

THE general divisions of Calisthenics embrace CHEST, SHOULDER, ELBOW, ARM AND HAND, HEAD AND NECK, TRUNK AND WAIST, KNEE, LEG AND FOOT, AND COMBINED EXERCISES.

It will be remembered that the execution of the following exercises is done by all the students simultaneously and equally, so that each position is taken and each motion is begun by all at the same moment, and each class of movements is executed in the same time, which is to be marked as described p. 14.

In executing the movements, the right side will have precedence of the left; the front of the rear. Movements to the sides will always precede correspondent ones to the front and rear.

ORAL ELEMENTS.

THE instructor will first require the students to pronounce a catch-word once, and then produce the oral element represented by the figured vowel, or *italic* consonant, four times—thus: àge, à, à, à, à; ăt, â, å, ä, ä, &c. He will exercise the class perseveringly, until each student can utter *consecutively* all of the elementary sounds, as arranged in the following

Table of Oral Elements.

I. TONICS.

à, as in àge.	ē, as in hē.	ŏ, as in ŏn.
ă, " ăt.	ĕ, " ĕnd.	ō, " dō.
ä, " ärt.	ê,³ " hêr.	u,⁴ " pure.
â, " âll.	ī, " īce.	ŭ, " ŭp.
à,¹ " bâre.	ĭ, " ĭt.	ü, " fůll.
ä,² " äsk.	ō, " ōld.	ou " our.

II. SUBTONICS.

b, as in bib.	m, as in maim.	v, as in vine.
d, " did.	n, " nine.	w, " will.
g, " gag.	ng, " sing.	y, " you.
j, " jib.	r,⁵ " rare.	z, " zest.
l, " lo.	ᴛʜ, " ᴛʜis.	z, " azure.

---

¹ **A Fifth.**—The *fifth* element, or sound, represented by *a*, is its *first* or *alphabetic* sound, modified or softened by *r*. In its production, the lips, placed nearly together, are held immovable while the student tries to utter the *first* or *alphabetic* sound of *a*

² **A Sixth.**—The *sixth* element represented by *a*, is a sound intermediate between *a* as heard in *at*, *ash*, and *a* as in *arm*, *art*. It is produced by prolonging and slightly softening *a* as heard in *at*.

³ **E Third.**—The *third* element represented by *e*, is *e* as heard in *end*, prolonged, and modified or softened by *r*.

⁴ **U Initial.**—*U*, at the beginning of words, when long, has the sound of *yu*, as in *use*.

⁵ **R Trilled.**—In *trilling r*, the tip of the tongue is made to vibrate rapidly against the roof of the mouth. The instructor will frequently require students, after a full inhalation, to trill *r* continuously, as long as possible. *R* may be trilled when immediately followed by a vowel.

III. ATONICS.

f, as in *f*ife.	*s*, as in *s*ense.	*sh*, as in *sh*y.
h, " *h*ill.	*t*, " *t*art.	*wh*,[1] " *wh*y.
k, " *k*ick.	*th*, " *th*in.	
p, " *p*ipe.	*ch*, " *ch*in.	

Students will also be required to form combinations by prefixing and affixing subtonics or atonics to the tonics. As the *fifth* element represented by *a*, and the *third* element of *e*, are always immediately followed by the oral element of *r* in words, the *r* should be introduced in like manner in the combinations. The *sixth* sound of *a* is always immediately followed by the oral element of *f*, *n*, or *s*, in the same syllable. For convenience, *f* only will be employed in combination.

1. Form the combinations by prefixing or affixing the subtonics to the tonics; as,

bā, bȧ, bä, bȧ, bär, bȧf; bē, bĕ, bêr;
bī, bĭ; bō, bò, bŏ; bū, bŭ, bu̇, bou.
ȧb, ȧb, ȧb, ȧb, ärb, ȧf; ĕb, &c.

2. Form the combinations by prefixing or affixing the atonics to the tonics; as,

fā, fȧ, fä, fȧ, fär, fȧf; fē, fĕ, fêr;
fī, fĭ; fō, fò, fŏ; fū, fŭ, &c.

3. Form the combinations by employing both subtonics and atonics with the tonics; as,

bāf, bȧf, bäf, bȧf, bär, bȧf; bēf, bĕf, &c.

RESPIRATION.

A SKILLFUL management of the respiratory organs while employing the voice, or during periods of muscular exertion, is of the utmost importance. When talking or read-

---

[1] **Wh.**—To produce the oral element of *wh*, the student will blow from the center of the mouth—first compressing the lips, and then suddenly relaxing them while the air is escaping.

ing, the breath should be drawn or gathered at the pauses, or *intervals* of the period, thus fully supplying the lungs with air, without improper interruptions. While taking calisthenic exercises, without employing the voice, the breathing, unless otherwise directed, should be carried on through the nose.

In order to enlarge and strengthen the lungs, and give depth, mellowness, and purity to the voice, the instructor will frequently combine the following respiratory exercises with the production of the elementary sounds of the language. The students will stand in an erect, but easy posture; the arms akimbo; the fingers pressed on the abdominal muscles, in front, and the thumbs on the dorsal muscles, on each side of the spine, as in Fig. 25, p. 60.

The action of the chest, the diaphragm, and the abdominal muscles will be free and unrestrained. The respiratory exercises will occasionally be executed in connection with appropriate music, or counting by the instructor.

1. DEEP BREATHING. Draw in and give out the breath, fully and slowly, eight times through the nose, and then eight times through the mouth, producing the prolonged sound of *h* on each exhalation from the mouth.

2. EXPLOSIVE BREATHING. Draw in a very full breath through the mouth, and emit it suddenly in a brief sound of the letter *k*, sixteen times. Rise on the toes with each inhalation, and recover the commencing position with each exhalation.

3. PANTING. Inhale and exhale sixteen times through the nose, and then sixteen times through the mouth. The inspiration and expiration must be very quick and violent, the expiration predominating in force and sound.

4. PRODUCE THE ATONICS in connection with calisthenic movements,—the instructor counting, when music is not employed. Each oral element will be uttered eight times, once on each motion from the position, the students audibly and fully inflating their lungs each time while recovering the commencing position.

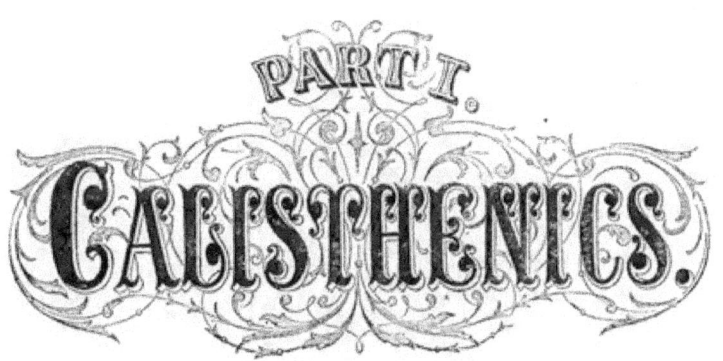

PART I.
CALISTHENICS.

CALISTHENICS.

CALISTHENIC exercises are arranged in this treatise chiefly for class drill in schools and families, and for the necessary preliminary lessons of the gymnasium. They, however, are adapted to the wants of all persons, either individually or in classes. Practiced systematically and sedulously, they will give development of muscular fiber, increased arterialization, and improved innervation, insuring the regulation of associated, and the equal development of antagonistic groups of muscles. While the classes of movements should always be executed in the prescribed order, they may be repeated at pleasure when employed as specifics.

To invigorate the respiratory system, expand the chest, and acquire an upright carriage, the student will frequently execute the following Chest, Shoulder, Elbow, and Arm and Hand Exercises—especially the movements of Nos. 4, 5, 6, 10, 14, 22, 23, 24, 25, 26, 40, 42, 43, 44, 46, 48, 54, 55, 56, 58, 61, 63, 67, 69, 70, 71, 76, 77, 97, 102, 124, 125, 193, 262, 263, 265, 266, 268, 269, 272, and 274. In cases of incipient consumption, the movements should often be described while the lungs are fully inflated.

The Trunk and Waist, Knee, Leg and Foot, and Combined Exercises are valuable in cases of dyspepsia and torpid liver, affording relief to constipated bowels, and frequently removing general muscular weakness. The most valuable classes of movements for dyspeptics are those of Nos. 142, 143, 144, 146, 149, 150, 151, 155, 156, 157, 159, 160, 161, 168, 169, 205, 206, 215, 218, 220, 322, 223, 230, 231, 232, 233, 241, 242, 243, 281, and 283.

I.

CHEST EXERCISE.[1]

FIRST SERIES.

First Position.

No. 1.—Immediately after the formation of the class, as is prescribed on p. 15, the instructor commands: 1. *Attention*—CLASS; 2. *Chest Exercise;* 3. *First Series;* 4. *First*—POSITION.

No. 2.—On hearing the *first* word of the first command, the students fix their *attention;* at the *second,* they always take the *habitual* or *military* position, p. 10, which brings the ear, shoulder, hip, knee, and ankle into line, as seen in Fig. 12.

No. 3.—When the fourth command is given, the students will take the first position, as represented by Fig. 13. The fists are placed together upon the breast, with their backs front, and the elbows are elevated *as high as the shoulders.*

No. 4.—*First Movements*—RIGHT. At this command, the students, marking time by counting,[2] or otherwise, as prescribed p. 14, will describe the arc A B, and recover the commencing position four times. The outward motions are the accented or more forcible ones. On the fourth outward motion the instructor will command, LEFT, when the students, as soon as they recover the commencing position, describe the arc C D four times. On the fourth outward motion with the left hand, the instructor commands, ALTERNATE, when the students, after recovering the commencing position, describe the arcs A B and C D alternately four times (twice to each arc), commencing with

---

[1] **Chest Exercise.**—As the first *three* classes of movements are made from and terminate with the chest, and all the movements from the *four* positions of this general division bring into play the chest-muscles, and as a more convenient classification is thus secured, the first general division is called *Chest Exercise;* though, in a strict classification, it would be termed *Elbow Exercise.*

[2] Music, PHONETICS, and other VOCAL EXERCISES to accompany the Movements, pp. 38 to 48.

the arc A B. At the command, BOTH, the arcs will be described four times simultaneously. It will be seen that these arcs are so described that, at their terminations B and D, the backs of the fists are to the rear.

No. 5.—*Second Movements*[1]—RIGHT. The remaining commands of this class of movements, and the number and order of the movements, are the same as in No. 4 ; but the motions are made from the first position directly out at the sides and behind, as far as possible, the arcs described being horizontal.

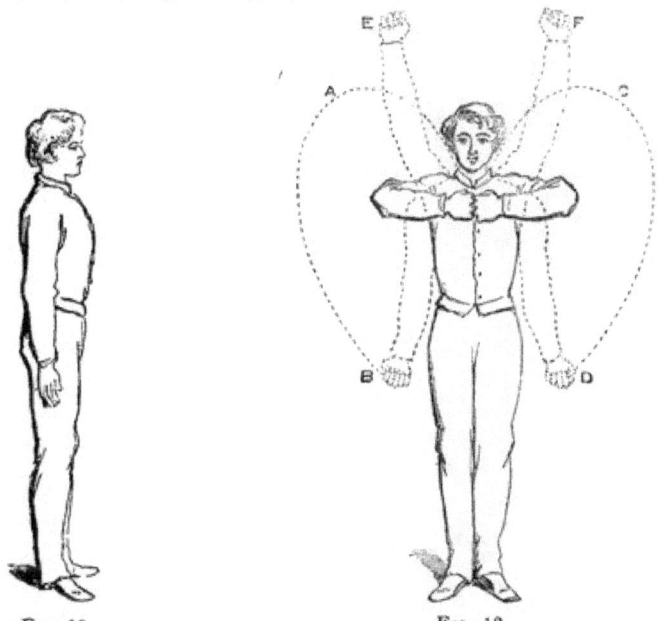

FIG. 12. FIG. 13.

No. 6.—*Third Movements*—RIGHT. The motions of this class are made up and off at an angle of 45 degrees from the first position. The number and order of the movements are the same as in No. 4. On reaching the points E and F, the arms will be straight, and the backs of the fists to the rear.

---

[1] **Second Movements.**—The great point in this class of movements is to hold the arms *perpendicular* to the body, and throw them backward as far and as violently as possible, thus stretching the collar-bone and flattening the shoulder-blades. This gives room to the lungs in front, enlarges the chest, and tends to cure round shoulders.

Second Position.

No. 7.—The instructor commands, *Second*—POSITION; and the students instantly, at the second word of command, place their elbows by their sides, in line with the waist, and their fists against their shoulders, backs front, as represented in Fig. 14.

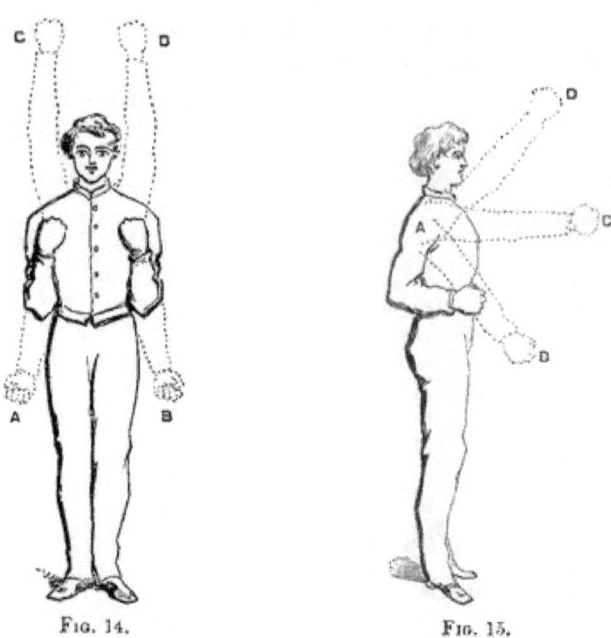

Fig. 14.   Fig. 15.

No. 8.—*First Movements*—RIGHT. At this command, the right forearm is carried directly down, as at A, Fig. 14, and returned to the commencing position four times; when, at the command, LEFT, four corresponding motions are made with the left forearm, terminating at B; then, at the command, ALTERNATE, four downward motions are made alternately; and finally, at the command, BOTH, four downward motions are described with both forearms simultaneously.

No. 9.—*Second Movements*—RIGHT. The remaining commands, and the number and order of the movements, are the same as in No. 8; but the motions are made directly front, by straightening the arms and recovering the commencing position.

CHEST EXERCISE.   35

No. 10.—*Third Movements*—Right. The number and order of these movements are the same as in No. 8. The movements are executed by thrusting the arms directly up as high as possible to the points C and D, Fig. 14.

Third Position.

No. 11.—At the command, *Third*—Position, the students take the position of Fig. 15, in which the forearms are placed against the waist, with the backs of the fists out to the sides.

No. 12.—There are three classes of movements from the third position: the first of which is described in the direction A B, Fig. 15; the second, in the direction A C; and the third, in the direction A D. The commands, and the number and order of the motions, are the same as those of the Second Position, p. 34.

Fourth Position.

No. 13.—At the command, *Fourth*—Position, the students place their fists back of and against their hips, with the backs of the hands out, the thumbs closed in front, and the elbows pressed down and toward each other, as represented in Fig. 16.

No. 14.—The first class of movements from this position is executed in the direction A B; the second, in the direction A C; and the third, by describing the arc E D. In executing the third class of movements, the body will maintain a position as nearly vertical as possible. The outward or upward motions, which are produced with great vigor, terminate only when the fists are as high as, and in line with, the shoulders at the point D. The commands, and the number and order of the motions, are the same as those of the Second Position, p. 34.

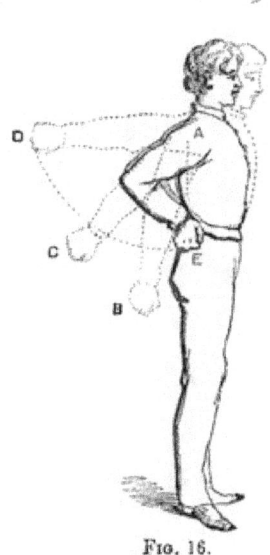

Fig. 16.

SECOND SERIES.

First Position.

No. 15.—The instructor will command: 1. *Chest Exercise;* 2. *Second Series;* 3. *First*—POSITION.

No. 16.—At the third command, the students will take the first position, as represented in Fig. 17. The backs of the fists are placed upon the breast, and the elbows are elevated as high as possible, preparatory to the movements.

No. 17.—The commands, the positions, the classes of movements, and the order, direction, and number of motions, are the same in the *Second Series* of Chest Exercises as in the *First*, with only the difference that the backs of the fists are always *within*, thus reversing the action of all the muscles.

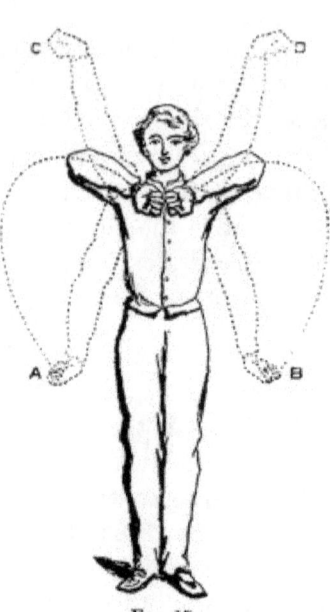

FIG. 17.

The positions of the backs of the hands, in all stages of execution of the movements of the FIRST SERIES, *must be reversed in the* SECOND.

THIRD SERIES.

First Position.

No. 18.—The instructor commands: 1. *Chest Exercise;* 2. *Third Series;* 3. *Positions of First* (or *Second*) *Series;* 4 *First* —POSITION.

No. 19.—The positions of the *Third Series* are the same as those of the *First Series,* or of the *Second,* in accordance with the part announced of the third preparatory command of No. 18. The students will take all of the positions in regular order, and execute a class of movements from each in combination, as follows: At the command, RIGHT, the right member describes the first motion of the first class of movements, and recovers the commencing position; the first of the second; the first of the third; and, again, the first of the second. At the command, LEFT, the left member executes the same number of corresponding motions; and, finally, at the command, BOTH, both members execute these motions simultaneously, and immediately repeat their execution. For example, the class of combined movements from the first position of Chest Exercise, Fig. 13, will be executed as follows: First, the right arm describes the arc A B, and recovers the commencing position; then it makes a motion directly back in line with the shoulder, and recovers the commencing position; then it is thrown up, like the dotted arm, E, and brought back to the commencing position; and, finally, the horizontal motion is repeated. The same number of corresponding motions is then made with the left arm. In conclusion, both arms execute these motions simultaneously, and immediately repeat their execution.

FOURTH SERIES.[1]

First Position.

No. 20.—The instructor commands: 1. *Chest Exercise;* 2. *Fourth Series;* 3. *First*—POSITION.

No. 21.—At the last command, the students take the first position, fists at A and B, as represented in Fig. 18.

No. 22.—*First Movements*—RIGHT. At the command, RIGHT, the students commence inhaling air; and on *one* (the instructor, or an assistant, does the counting, or otherwise marks the time), they simultaneously strike the right lung smartly, near the lower ribs, with the right fist; on *two*, the hand recovers its commencing position at A; on *three*, the fist is struck against the lung immediately above the

---

[1] **Fourth Series.**—The exercises of this series tend to expand the lungs and increase the flexibility of all the muscles of the chest, and those of the abdominal and dorsal region which are concerned in respiration. They are among the best preventives of consumption.

previous place ; and so the right fist advances upward until, on *seven*, the right lung is struck just below the clavicle, or collar-bone, when the command, LEFT, is given, and the left lung is struck four times in like manner with the left fist. At the command, ALTERNATE, the lungs are struck alternately four times, when the instructor commands, BOTH, and the lungs are struck simultaneously, with both fists, four times.

No. 23.—*Second Movements*—RECIPROCATE. At this command, from the first position of Fig. 18, the student, on *one*, strikes the left lung near the lower ribs with the right fist ; on *two*, the right fist recovers the commencing position, and the left one gives a corresponding blow to the right lung ; on *three*, the left fist recovers its commencing position, and the right one strikes the left lung just above the previous place. These reciprocating motions continue until, on *eight*, the left fist strikes the right lung just below the collar-bone, when the direction of the beating is reversed, and terminates with the lower ribs on the *second eight*. An immediate repetition of this beating up and down the chest completes the second class of movements from the first position. These movements should be executed with great rapidity.

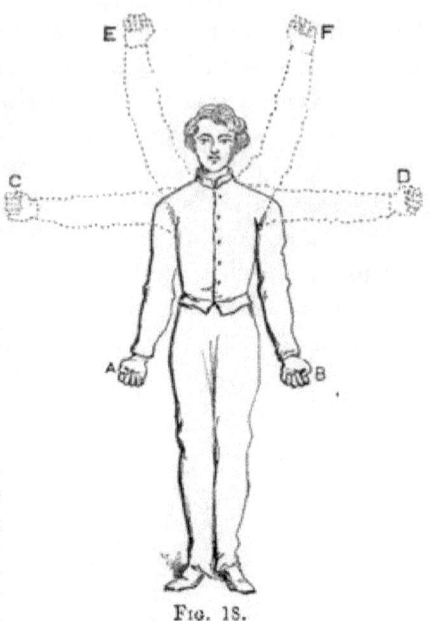

FIG. 18.

No. 24.—During the execution of these movements, the students will take deep inspirations, retaining the air in the lungs, when fully inflated, as long as possible, and then let the breath go out steadily and slowly, not permitting the air, however, to become completely exhausted at any time. Both the inspiration and expiration are done through the nose, the mouth remaining closed. The lungs are beaten smartly from the lower ribs up to the collar-bone ; but *the middle of the chest is not struck.*

Second Position.

No. 25.—At the command, *Second*—POSITION, the students stretch the arms out sidewise as high as the shoulders, with the fists at c and D, Fig. 18. The remaining commands, and the classes of movements from this position, are the same as those of the first position.

Third Position.

No. 26.—*Third*—POSITION. At this command, the arms will be so elevated as to place the fists at E and F, Fig. 18. The commands and the classes of movements are the same as those given from the first position; but the direction of the beating is reversed, commencing with the collar-bone.

No. 27.—The instructor will frequently require the class *in review* to take the positions and execute the movements of an entire series of exercises without words of command. In that event, *on the last accented motion of each class of movements, the students will take the position next in order, instead of resuming the commencing position.*

VOCAL EXERCISES.

Varieties.

IN combining vocal exercises with Calisthenics, as is prescribed on p. 14, the instructor will employ only such varieties as are best adapted to the exercises under consideration at the time. A great variety is here introduced, for convenient reference.

I. COUNTING.

No. 28.—The figures employed for indices show the number of motions that are made before one of the *four* general changes of a class of movements occurs. The motions from given positions are indicated by odd numbers, and those to recover commencing positions by even ones. The heavy or accented syllables are indicated by accented vowels. They are prolonged or dwelt upon twice as long as light or unaccented syllables. The students count continuously from *one* to *eight*, inclusive, naming each number once, twice, or three times. To afford a greater variety, the class will occasionally sing the numbers, letting the voice rise and fall in regular progression, as in singing the musical scale.

1st. óne, twó, thrée, fóur, fíve, síx, séven, éight; &c.

2d. óne one, twó two, thrée three, fóur four, fíve five, síx six, séven seven, éight eight; óne one, twó two, thrée three, &c.

3d. one óne, two twó, three thrée, four fóur, five fíve, &c.

4th. óne one one, twó two two, thrée three three, fóur four four, fíve five five, síx six six, séven seven seven, éight eight eight; &c.

5th. one óne one, two twó two, three thrée three, &c.

6th. one one óne, two two twó, three three thrée, &c.

II. PHONETICS.

No. 29.—The indices and the marks of accent are employed for the same purpose as in No. 28. The combinations of the tonics with the subtonics and the atonics are given on the *twenty-eighth* p. The students will commence with the first oral element of *a*, and give the tonics *consecutively* as arranged in the Table of Oral Elements, p. 26, uttering each one the number of times indicated in the following exercises. The tonics will also be uttered consecutively *in combination*, as illustrated by the *eighth* variety of this section.

1st. á', ă', ä', â', âr', âf', ĕ', ĕ'; ĕr', ĭ', ĭ', ŏ', ŏ', ŏ', ŭ', ŭ'; &c.

                1   2   3   4   5   6   7   8   1
2d.   ă′ă, ă′ă, ă′ă, ă′ă, ȧr′ȧr, âf′âf, ĕ′ĕ, ĕ′ĕ; ẽr′ẽr, &c.

                1   2   3   4   5   6   7   8   1
3d.   ă ă′, ă ă′, ă ă′, ă ă′, ȧr ȧr′, âf âf′, ĕ ĕ′, ĕ ĕ′; ẽr ẽr′, &c.

                1   2   3   4   5   6
4th. ă′ă ă, ă′ă ă, ă′ă ă, ă′ă ă, ȧr′ȧr ȧr, âf′âf âf, &c.

                1   2   3   4   5   6
5th. ă ă′ă, ă ă′ă, ă ă′ă, ă ă′ă, ȧr ȧr′ȧr, âf âf′âf, &c.

                1   2   3   4   5   6
6th. ă ă ă′, ă ă ă′, ă ă ă′, ă ă ă′, ȧr ȧr ȧr′, âf âf âf′, &c.

         1 2 3 4 5 6 7 8   1 2 3 4 5 6 7 8
7th. ă′, ă′, ă′, ă′, ă′, ă′, ă′, ă′; ă′, ă′, ă′, ă′, ă′, ă′, ă′, ă′; &c.

                1   2   3   4   5   6   7   8
8th. brăch, brăch, brăch, brăch, brăch, brăch, brăch, brăch;
                1   2   3   4   5   6   7   8
        brăr, brăr, brăf, brăf, brĕch, brĕch, brĕch, brĕch;
                1   2   3   4   5   6
        brĕr, brĕr, brĭch, brĭch, brĭch, brĭch, &c.

III. RECITATIONS.

No. 30.—Marks of accent and indices are employed for the same purpose as in No. 28. For remarks on *recitations* and *songs* in connection with Calisthenics, see p. 14.

                1   2   3   4
1st.   Chárging, thén the cóursers springing—
                5   6   7   8
        Swórd and hélmet cláshing, rínging.

                1   2   3   4
2d.   He túgged, he shóok, till dówn it cáme—
                5   6   7   8
        The róof, the dóme, one shéet of fláme

3d.
   1   2   3   4
Háil to the chíef who in tríumph ad vánces ;
   5   6   7   8
Hónored and blést be the évergreen pine!

4th.
   1   2   3   4
The bóok is compléted, our lábor is éndęd,
   5   6   7   8
And énvy deféated, while lóve is defénded.

5th.
   1   2   3   4
May I góv ern my pás sions with áb solute swáy ;
   5   6   7   8
And grow wis er and bét ter as life wears awáy.

IV. Vocal Music.

No. 31.—The same varieties of measure and accent will be employed in singing songs as in recitation, see No. 30. The simplest form of combining vocal music and Calisthenics is by employing either the tonics, or the syllables of the gamut as follows:

   1 2 3 4 5 6 7 8 1 2 3 4 5 6 7 8
1st. dó, ré, mí, fá, sól, lá, sí, dó ; dó, sí, lá, sól, fá, mí, ré, dó.

   1 2 3 4 5 6 7 8 1
2d. dó do, ré re, mí mi, fá fa, sól sol, lá la, sí si, dó do ; dó do, &c.

   1 2 3 4 5 6 7 8 1
3d. do dó, re ré, mi mí, fa fá, sol sól, la lá, si sí, do dó ; do dó, &c.

   1 2 3 4 5 6
4th. dó do do, ré re re, mí mi mi, fá fa fa, sól sol sol, lá la la, &c.

   1 2 3 4 5 6
5th. do dó do, re ré re, mi mí mi, fa fá fa, sol sól sol, la lá la, &c.

   1 2 3 4 5 6
6th. do do dó, re re ré, mi mi mí, fa fa fá, sol sol sól, la la lá, &c.

INSTRUMENTAL MUSIC.

THE music here introduced is specially arranged for this work from the choicest productions of the ablest masters. It affords a sufficient variety for the entire course of calisthenic and gymnastic drill. The instructor, however, will not be confined to it; as nearly all marches, dances, and other pieces of music that are employed to secure simultaneous movements, are appropriate.

General Commands.

No. 32.—After students learn to recognize promptly the *four* commands given below, the instructor may dispense with vocal commands during a prescribed course of drill. The students will be taught to follow the order of the general divisions as given on p. 25, without words of command. All variations desired may be explained before the exercise commences.

I. ATTENTION.

No. 33.—Whenever the instructor wishes to commence the instruction; to make an important explanation; to vary the exercises, or secure marked attention for any purpose; he will command, *Attention*—CLASS; or, in music, *Attention*—ATTENTION. At the *first* word of the command, the students will fix their attention; at the *second*, they will take their standings and assume the *military* position. If the instructor wishes simply to secure the attention of the class, without a change of position, he will omit the second word of command, or one half of the music that is employed for the command.

Attention——ATTENTION.

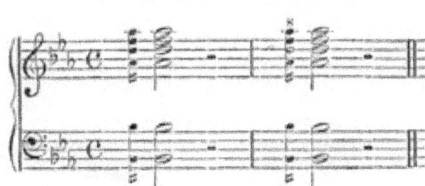

II. Position.

No. 34.—The commands for positions to be taken, when given in music, vary from the usual commands. The signal for POSITION, is first given; then the *number* of the position is announced by the number of times the next chord* is struck; and finally, the command, POSITION, is repeated, when the students take the position commanded.

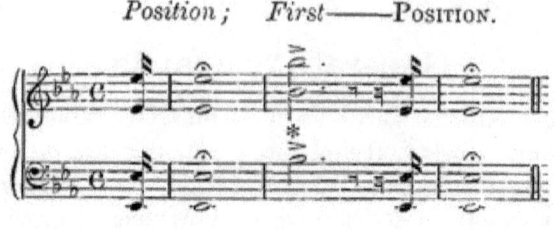

*Position;   First——*POSITION.

III. Movements.

No. 35.—The order of the commands for the Movements is reversed in music. For example, the command, *First—Movements*, becomes *Movements—First;* a rest being given between the two words of command. It will be seen that the repetition of the last two notes in the first command under this title, forms the second command. These two notes will be struck *three* times for *Third Movements; four* times for *Fourth*, &c. Immediately after this command, the piece of music for the Series of exercises under consideration will be performed, and the class of movements commanded will be executed in due order.

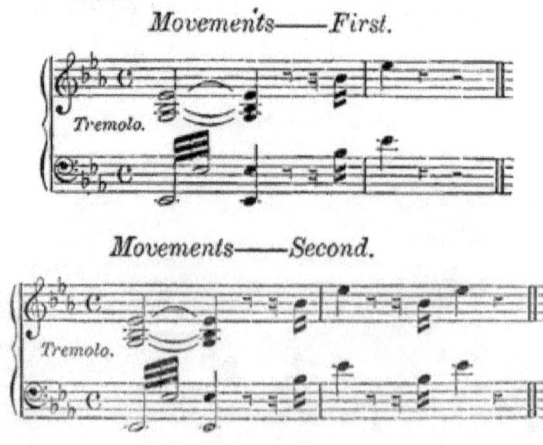

Movements——First.

Movements——Second.

IV. REST.

No. 36.—If the instructor wishes the class to rest without deranging the lines, he commands, *In place*—REST; or, in music, *Rest*—REST. At the last part of the command, each student, keeping his right foot on the line, will carry the left foot six inches to the rear, slightly bending the advanced knee, and let the weight of the body fall mainly on the foot in the rear. Then he will not be required to give attention, or preserve steadiness of position. If, on the contrary, the instructor should wish to rest the students without constraining them to preserve perfect lines, he will command, REST; or, in music, *Rest*—AS YOU PLEASE. At the last part of this command, they will not be required to preserve immobility, or to maintain their positions. They will not, however, entirely break up the ranks; but be in a position to instantly resume their standings at the command, ATTENTION.

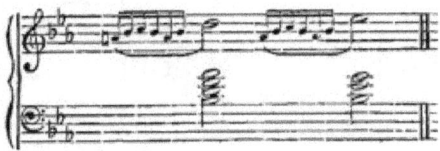

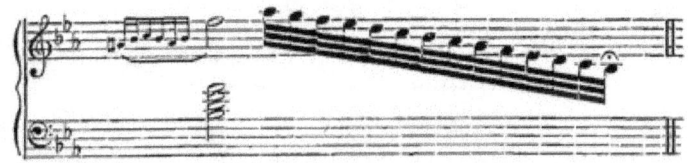

No. 37.—When music is employed in connection with Calisthenics or Gymnastics, *each piece will be repeated as often as required*. For example, the first piece of music that immediately follows, entitled "Part First of Chest Exercise," may be repeated *at pleasure*, answering for all the movements of each Series of that general division. In order to give variety, however, the instructor will use Part First for the First Series of Exercises; Part Second for the Second Series; Part First for the Third Series, &c.; or the two pieces of music may be used alternately, *the change occurring every time a new position is taken*.

CHEST EXERCISE.

PART FIRST.

Allegretto. VERDI.

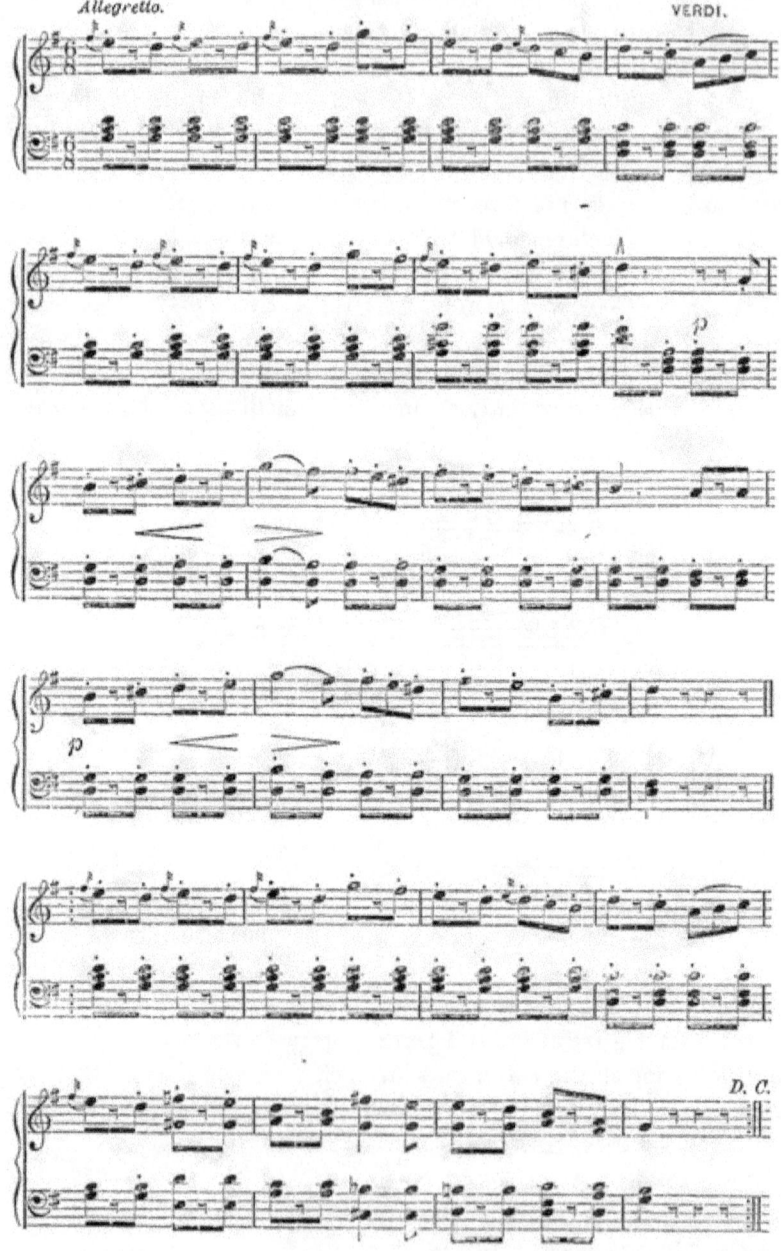

CHEST EXERCISE.

PART SECOND.

J. KUFFNER.

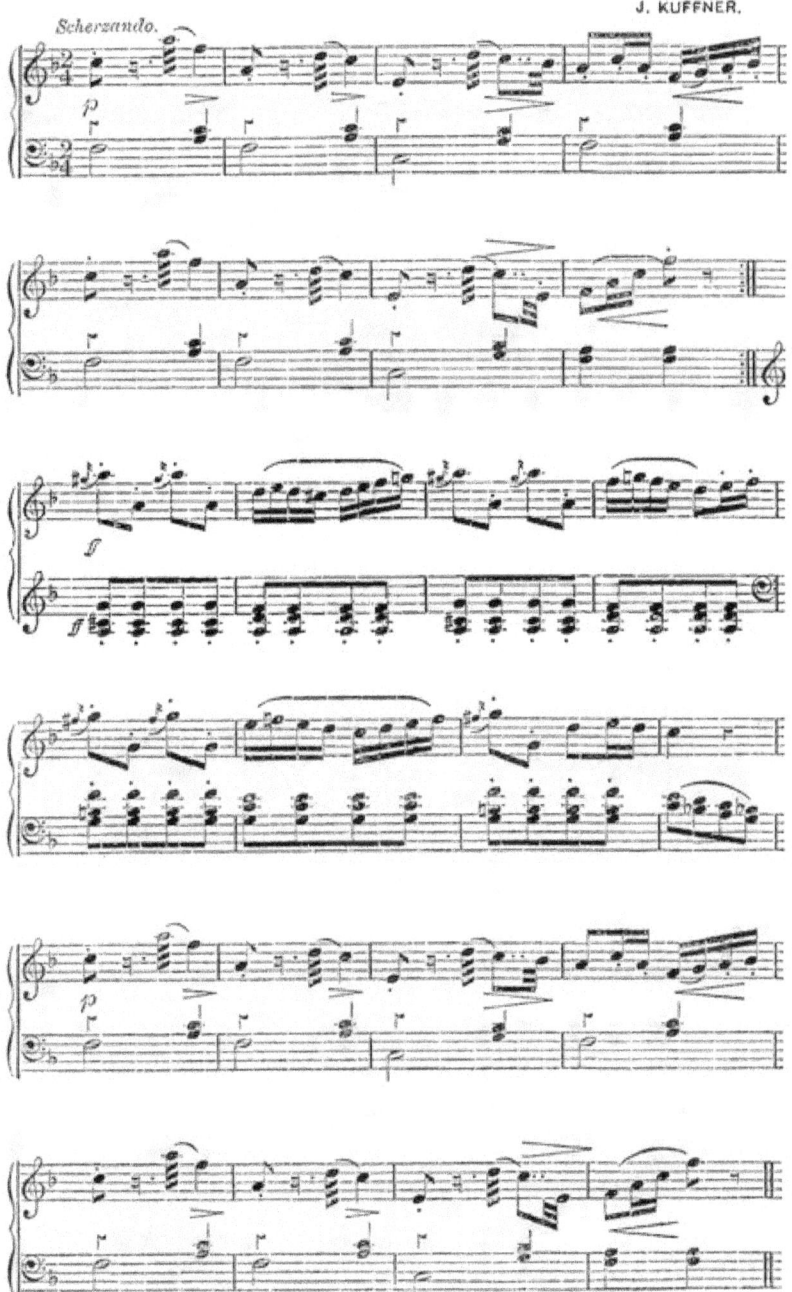

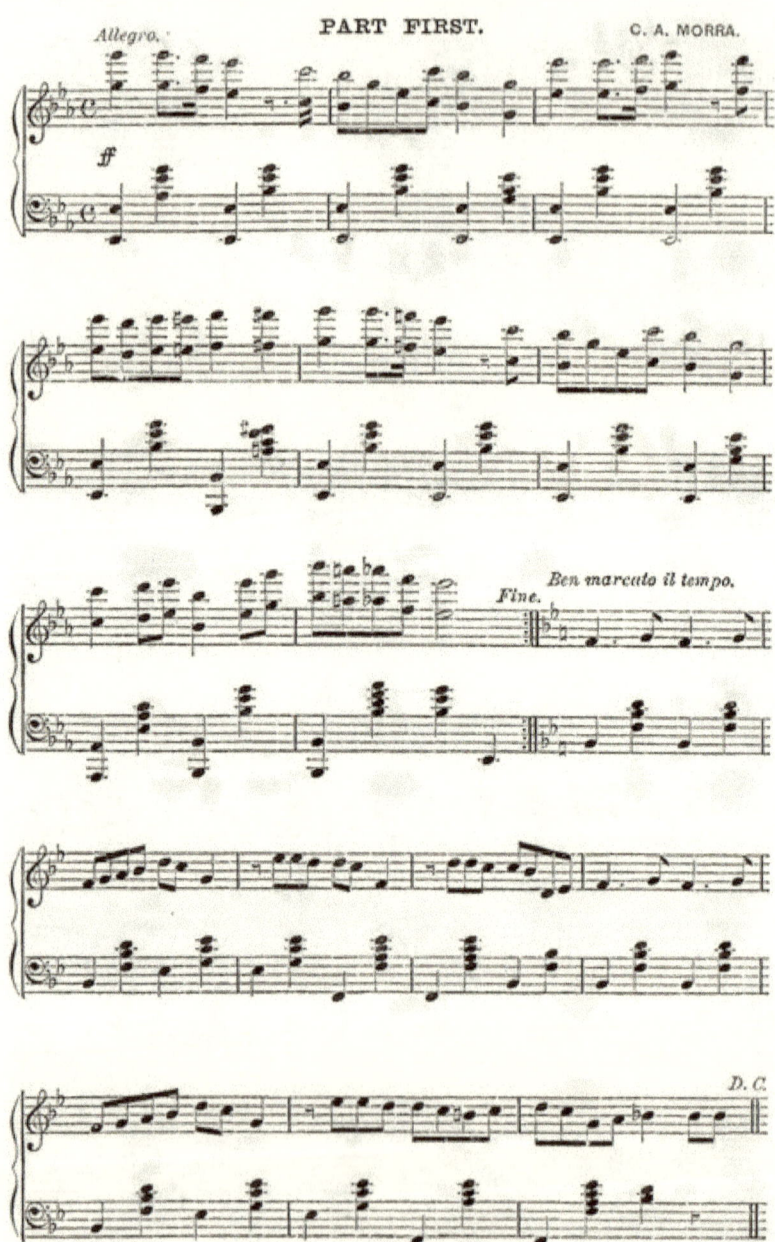

PART SECOND.

G. MEYERBEER.

Tempo di marcia, molto maestoso.

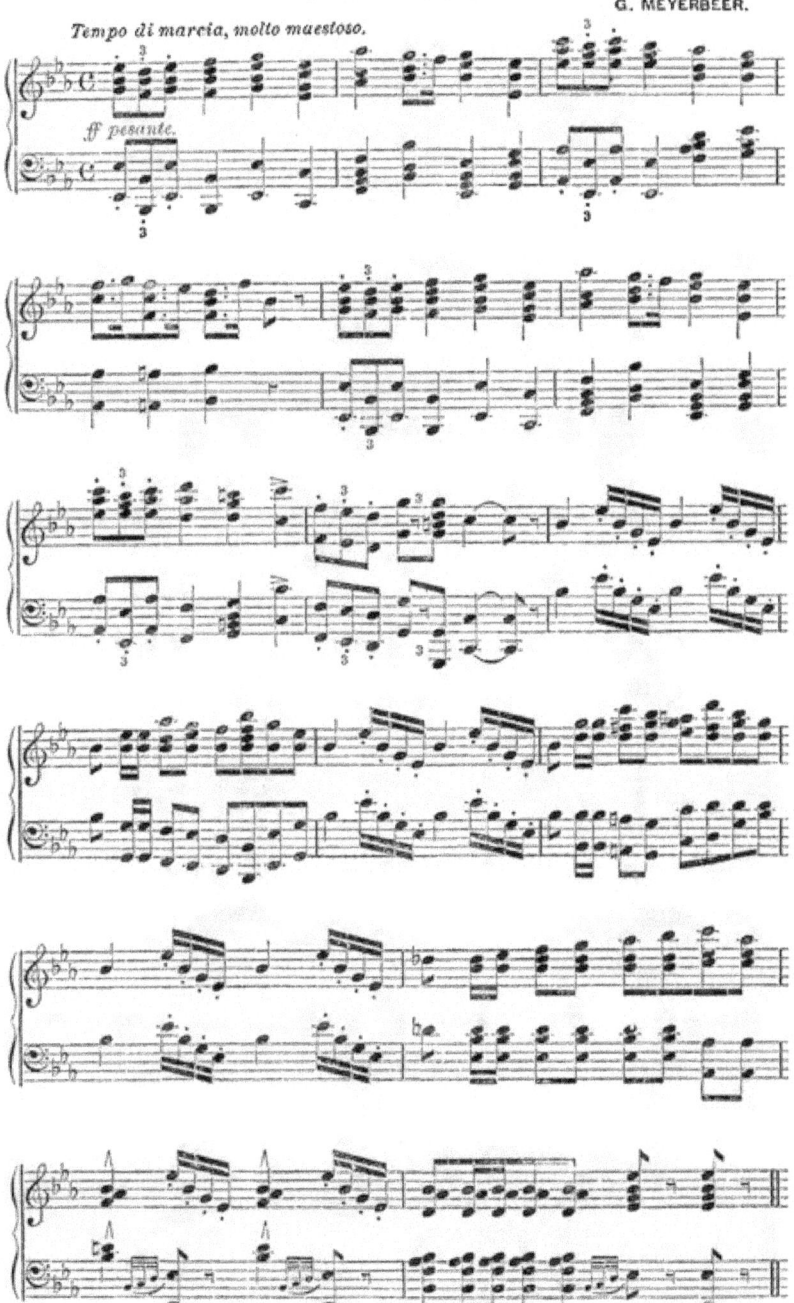

50   CALISTHENICS.

II.

SHOULDER EXERCISE.

FIRST SERIES.

First Position.

No. 38.—The instructor will command: 1. *Shoulder Exercise;* 2. *First Series;* 3. *First*—Position.[1]

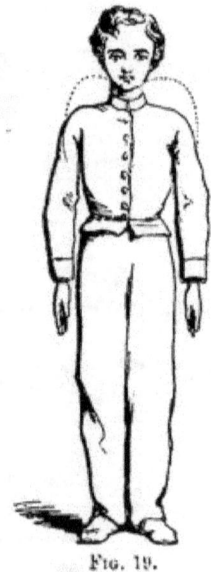

Fig. 19.

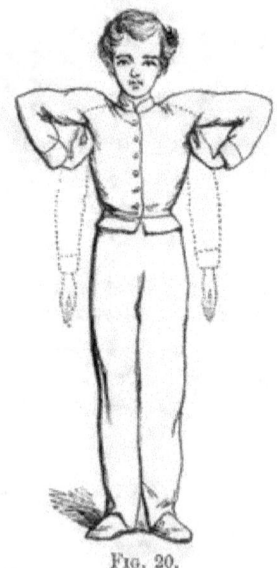

Fig. 20.

No. 39.—At the last word of the third command, the students take the first position, Fig. 19, which differs only from the *military*

---

[1] **First Position.**—The class of movements from this position brings into play the muscles which raise the shoulders and the upper ribs, and enlarges upward the cavity of the chest. It is of great service in cases of *incipient consumption,* and in partial *paralyzation of the shoulder muscles.* In cases of unequal height of the shoulders, proceeding from a partial paralyzation of one of them, or from the curvature of the spine, this movement should be performed frequently with the defective shoulder.

position in turning the elbows out a little and bringing the palms of the hands in, so that the thumbs point front.

No. 40.—The remaining commands are: 1. RIGHT; 2. LEFT; 3. ALTERNATE; 4. BOTH. At the first of these commands, the right shoulder is raised and lowered four times; at the second, the same number of corresponding motions is made with the left shoulder; at the third, these motions are made alternately four times, the right shoulder being first raised and lowered; and at the last command, both shoulders are raised together and lowered four times, as represented by the dotted lines of Fig. 19. During these movements, the arms are kept straight by the sides, the elbows remain unbent, and the shoulders are raised as powerfully and as high as possible. They must be lowered gently, that the head may not be too much shaken.

Second Position.

No. 41.—The instructor commands, *Second*—POSITION; and the students instantly take the position of Fig. 20, by raising the elbows at the sides as high as the shoulders, and placing the hands in the armpits with the thumbs front.

No. 42. —— *First Movements*——RIGHT. At this command, the right arm and hand are carried directly down, and returned to the commencing position four times, as represented in Fig. 20; when, at the command, LEFT, the left arm and hand execute the same number of corresponding motions; then, at the command, ALTERNATE, four downward motions are made alternately; and finally, at the command, BOTH, four downward motions are executed with both arms simultaneously.

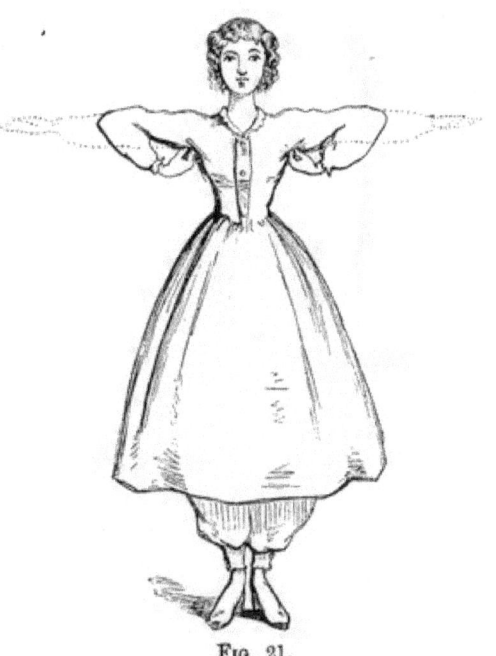

FIG. 21.

No. 43.—*Second Movements*—Right. The remaining commands, and the number and order of the movements, are the same as No. 42; but the motions are made directly out sidewise, as represented in Fig. 21.

No. 44.—*Third Movements*—Right. The number and order of these movements are the same as those of No. 42. The movements are executed by carrying the arms out sidewise; but, instead of having them terminate when the arms are straight, as represented in Fig. 21, they are continued until the arms are held vertical in line with the head, the backs of the hands being toward each other.

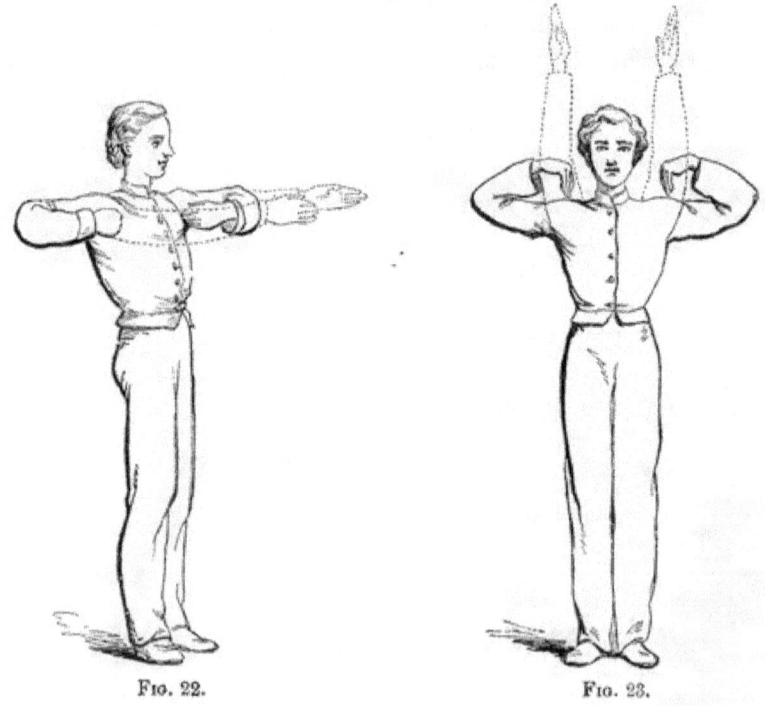

Fig. 22.   Fig. 23.

Third Position.

No. 45.—*Third*—Position. At this command, the points of the fingers are placed against the shoulders in front, where the arms and shoulders join, with the thumbs up and the elbows in line with the shoulders, as represented in Fig. 22.

No. 46.—The remaining commands, and the number and order of the movements from this position, are the same as from the second position; but the first class of movements is executed in front, as represented in Fig. 22; the second, by carrying the forearm directly out sidewise in line with the breast; and the third, by straightening the arms, and carrying them back horizontally as far as possible.

Fourth Position.

No. 47.—*Fourth*—POSITION. At this command, the points of the fingers are placed upon the shoulders where the arms and shoulders join, with the thumbs back, and the elbows in line with the shoulders, as in Fig. 23.

No. 48.—The commands, and the number and order of the movements from this position, are the same as from the second position; but the first class of movements is executed directly up, as represented in Fig. 23; the second, by keeping the elbows in position, and carrying the forearms directly sidewise; and the third, by straightening the arms and carrying them sidewise completely down against the thighs, with the hands open and the thumbs pointing back.

SECOND SERIES.

First Position.

No. 49.—The instructor commands: 1. *Shoulder Exercise;* 2. *Second Series;* 3. *First*—POSITION.

No. 50.—At the command, POSITION, the students will take the position of Fig. 20, which is the first position of the *Second Series.* The *second* position is the position of Fig. 22; the *third*, of Fig. 23.

No. 51.—The students will take these three positions in regular order, and execute one class of movements from each *in combination,* as follows: At the command, RIGHT, the right arm describes the first motion of the first class of movements, and recovers the commencing position; the first, of the second; the first, of the third; and again, the first of the second. At the command, LEFT, the left arm executes the same number of corresponding motions; and, finally, at the command, BOTH, both arms execute these motions simultaneously, and immediately repeat their execution. The movements of this series correspond to those of No. 19.

ELBOW EXERCISE.

PART FIRST.

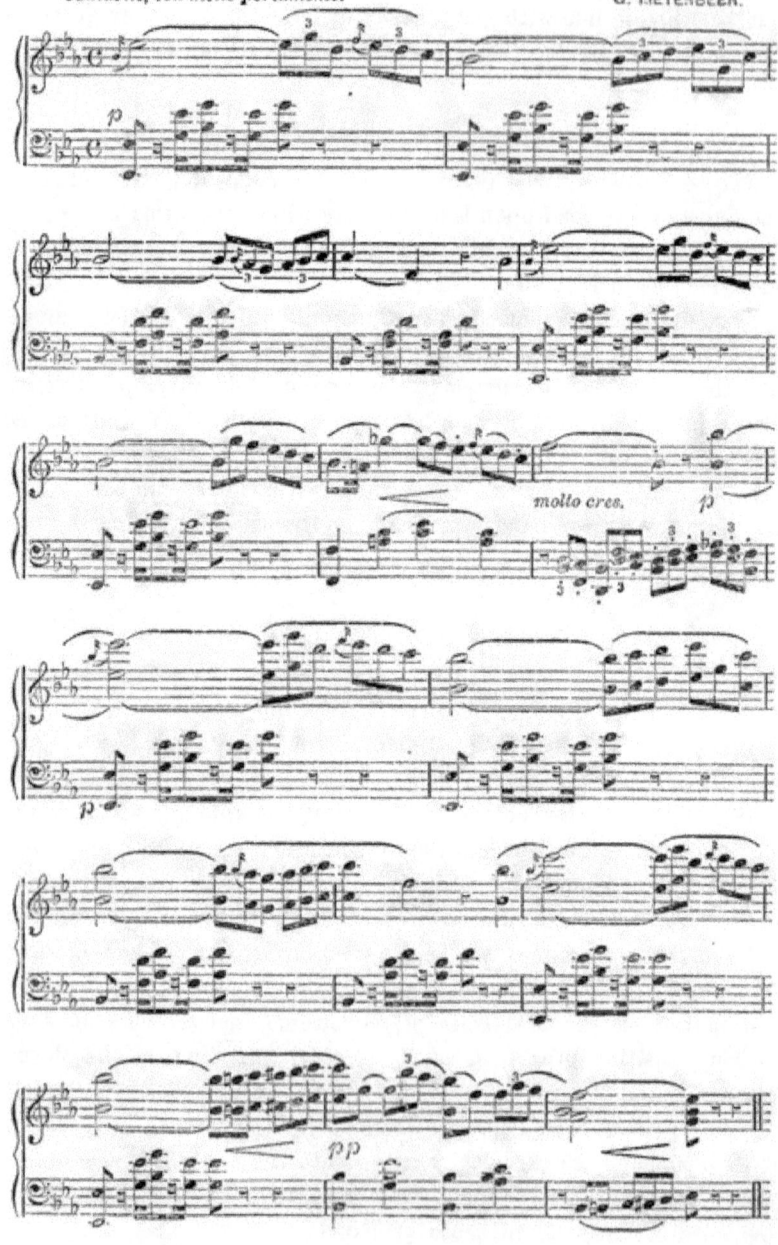

ELBOW EXERCISE.

PART SECOND.

DONIZETTI.

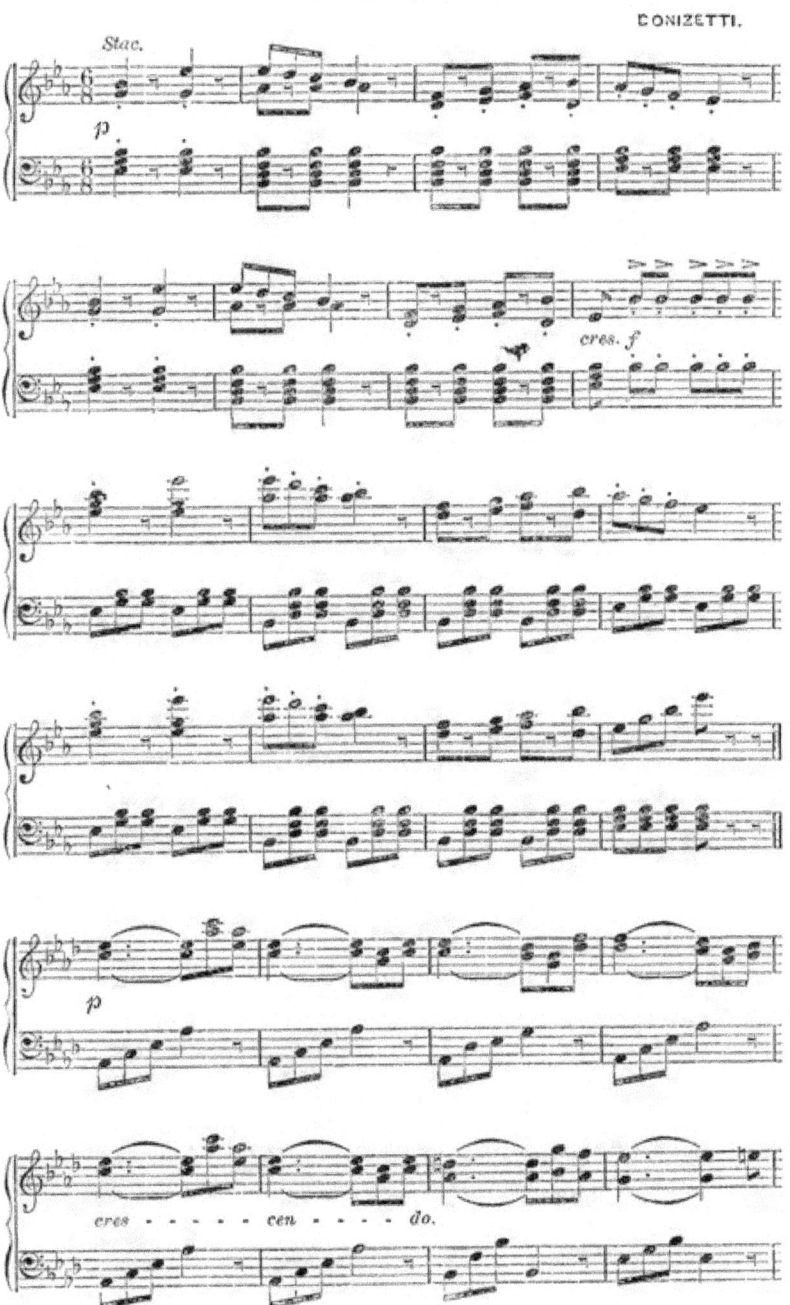

CALISTHENICS.

ARM AND HAND EXERCISE.

PART FIRST.

G. MEYERBEER.

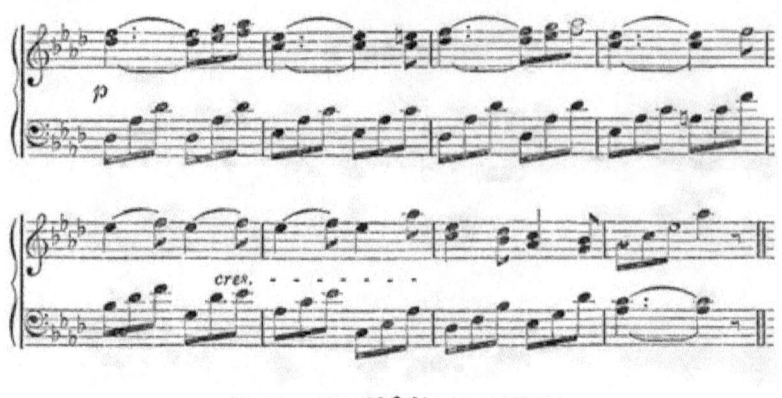

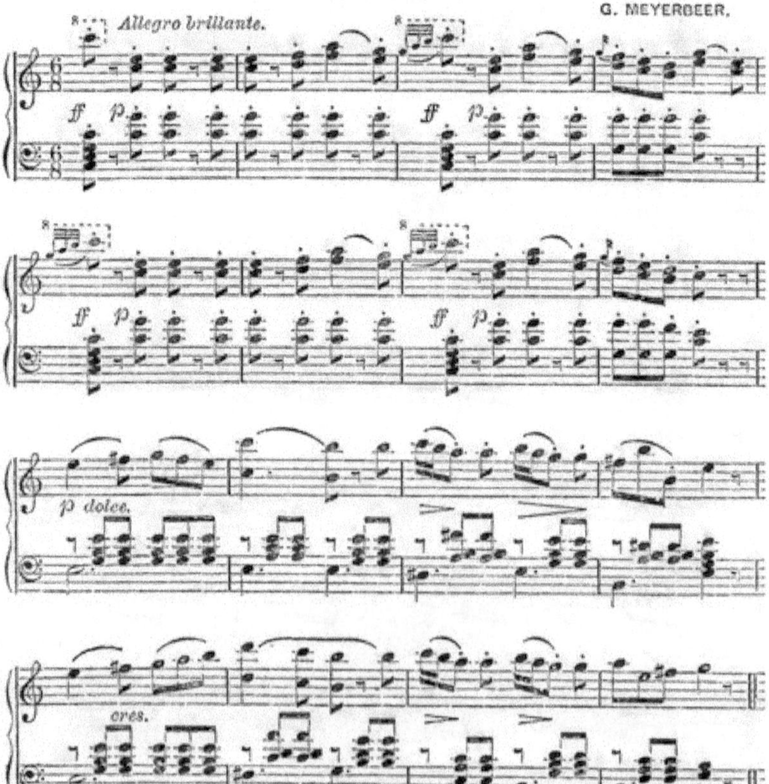

ARM AND HAND EXERCISE.

PART SECOND.

JAS. BELLAK.

PART THIRD.

STRAUSS.

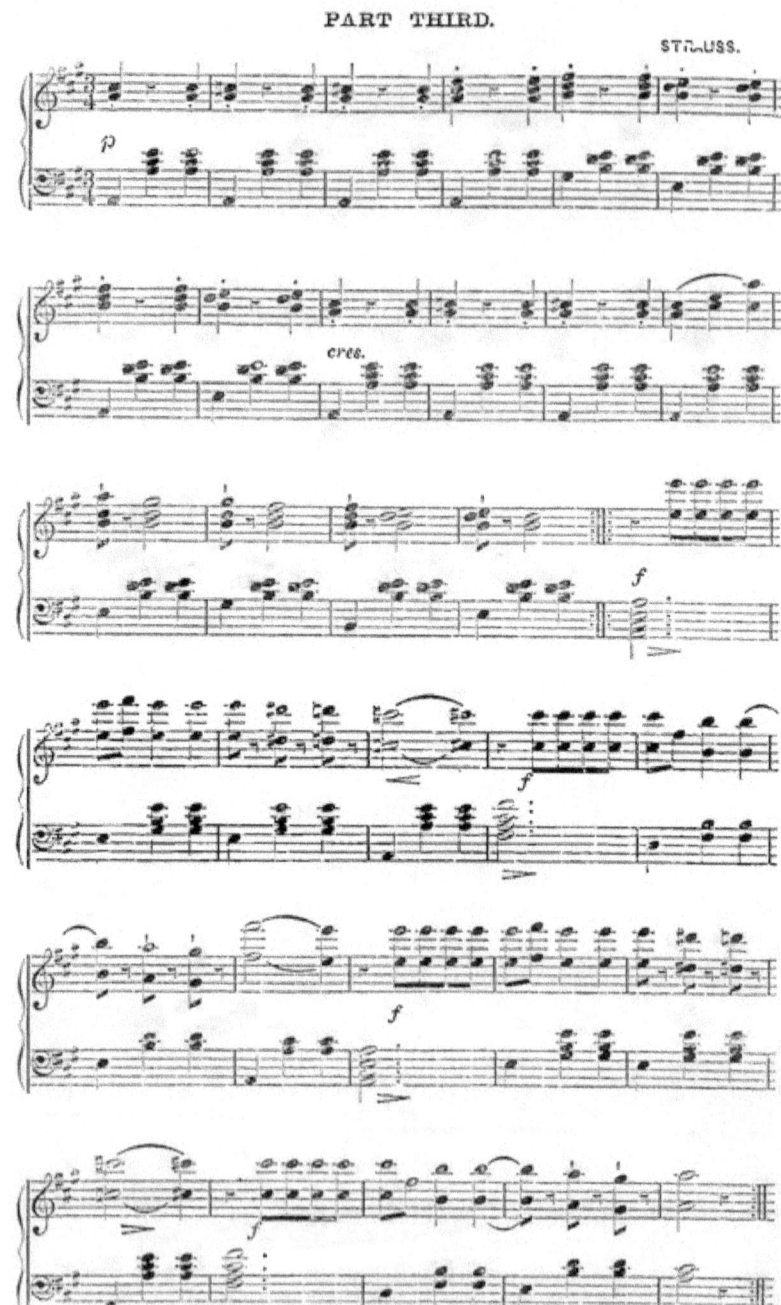

III.

ELBOW EXERCISE.

FIRST SERIES.

First Position.

No. 52.—The instructor will command: 1. *Elbow Exercise;* 2. *First Series;* 3. *First*—POSITION.

No. 53.—At the last command, the students will take the position of Fig. 24, which is the same as the first position of Chest Exercise, No. 3.

No. 54.—*First Movements*—RIGHT. At this command, the students will force the right elbow down and back, *as far as possible,* at an angle of 45 degrees, as represented by the lower dotted elbows of Fig. 24, and recover the commencing position four times. At the command, LEFT, the left elbow will execute a corresponding motion and recover the commencing position four times; when, at the command, ALTERNATE, four corresponding motions from the commencing position will be executed by the elbows alternately; after which, at the command, BOTH, four of these motions from the commencing position will be executed by both elbows simultaneously. *In executing these movements, the fists must be drawn from the breast, without varying the bend of the elbow.*

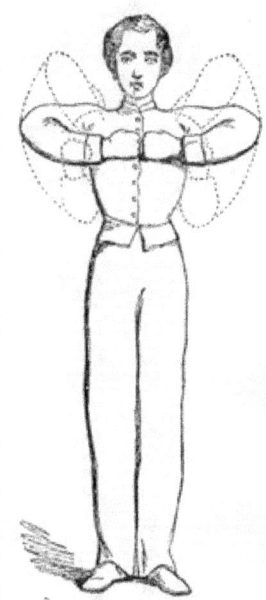

FIG. 24.

No. 55.—*Second Movements*—RIGHT. The remaining commands, and the number and order of the movements of this class, are the same as No. 54; but the motions are made with the elbows directly back from the position of Fig. 24, as far as possible. Read the note on p. 33, which is equally applicable to this class of movements.

No. 56.—*Third Movements*—RIGHT. The motions of this class are described directly up and out, *as far as possible,* at an angle of

45 degrees, as represented by the upper dotted elbows of Fig. 24. The number and order of the movements are the same as in No. 54.

Second Position.

No. 57.—The instructor commands, *Second*—POSITION; and the students take the position of Fig. 25, in which the hands are set fast on the hips, with the thumbs back.

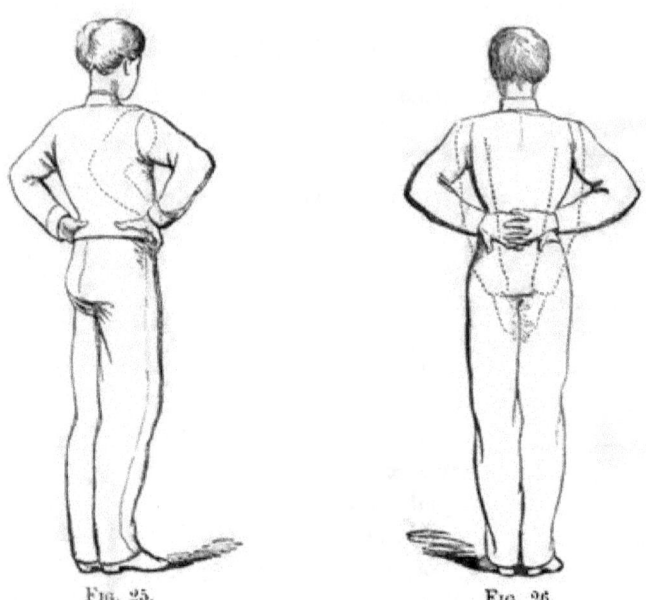

Fig. 25.   Fig. 26.

No. 58.—*First Movements*—RIGHT. The class of movements from this position is executed by first throwing the right elbow forcibly back, see dotted arm of Fig. 25, and recovering the commencing position, four times; then the left elbow describes four corresponding motions; then four like motions are made with the elbows by alternation; and, finally, four motions are made by both elbows simultaneously.

Third Position.[1]

No. 59.—At the command, *Third*—POSITION, the students take

---

[1] **Third Position.**—By the movements from the third position, the shoulders are strengthened, thrown more back and drawn down, thereby widening the chest and promoting a nobler carriage. *A valuable addition*

the position by interlacing the fingers, and placing the hands firmly against the small of the back, thumbs pointing down, as in Fig. 26.

No. 60.—*First Movements*—RIGHT. The first class of movements from this position is the same as No. 58.

No. 61.—*Second Movements*—DOWN. At this command, keeping the body perfectly vertical, the hands are thrust down as far as possible, and returned to the commencing position four times, as in Fig. 26; then, at the command, UP, an arc is described in the rear, by thrusting the hands and arms back and up, as high as possible, and resuming the commencing position four times; and finally, at the command, ALTERNATE, eight motions are made alternately from the commencing position,—the first being *down*, and the second, *back* and *up*.

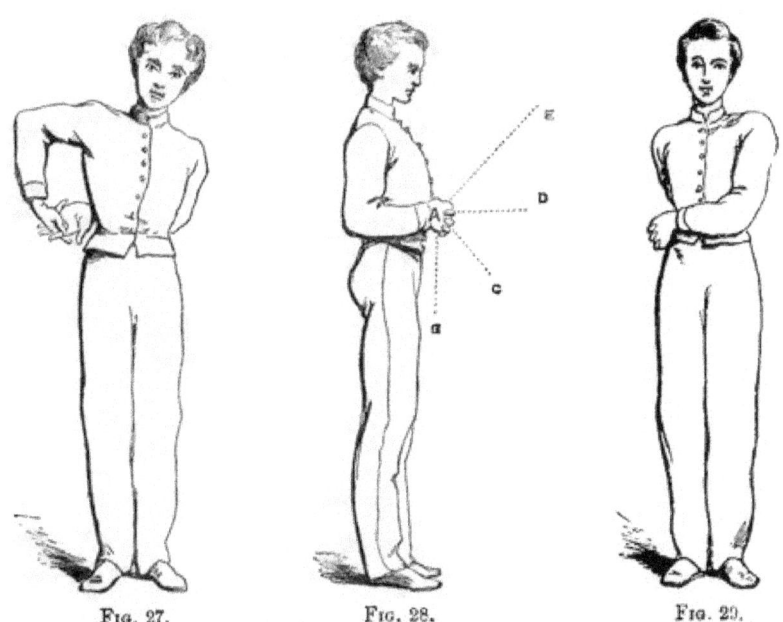

FIG. 27.   FIG. 28.   FIG. 29.

No. 62.—*Third Movements*—RIGHT. At this command, the knit hands are passed, in line with the waist, from the third position

---

to these movements may be secured by requiring the students to exhale the breath on every motion from the posi- tion, and to inhale fresh air every time the position is resumed, executing the movements slowly.

to the right side, in such a manner as to draw the left arm firmly against the left side and across the spine, showing the hands in front, as represented in Fig. 27, when the commencing position is resumed. This movement is made four times to the right; four times to the left; four times from the commencing position by alternation to the right and left: and at the command, BOTH, eight motions are made completely round from side to side,—the first motion commencing from, and the eighth terminating with, the commencing position.

Fourth Position.

No. 63.—The instructor commands, *Fourth*—POSITION, and the students take the position by placing the clasped hands against the abdomen, with their backs front, the elbows being so bent as to form right angles, as in Fig. 28.

No. 64.—*First Movements*—RIGHT. This class of movements corresponds to the movements of No. 57; but the motions from the commencing position are made directly front with the elbows, the hands retaining their position.

No. 65.—*Second Movements*—DOWN. At this command, the arms are stretched directly down as far as possible, the clasped hands describing the line A B in Fig. 28, and brought back to the commencing position four times; four outward motions are then made in the line A D; and, finally, eight outward motions are made alternately in the lines A B and A D. At the termination of each outward motion of this class, and the one immediately following, the palms will be brought forcibly together, thus producing sounds by the concussion which mark the time.

No. 66.—*Third Movements*—FRONT. The number and order of these movements correspond to those of No. 65; but the motions are made in the lines A C and A E.

No. 67.—*Fourth Movements*—RIGHT. The number and order of these movements correspond to those of No. 61; but the motions are made from the fourth position by carrying the hands to the side and back, as in Fig. 29. Throw hands behind much farther than represented in this figure. The face and the feet are to be kept forward. This class of movements is very important in strengthening the abdominal muscles. It should be performed with great force, but not fast.

ELBOW EXERCISE. 63

Fifth Position.

No. 68.—At the command, *Fifth*—POSITION, the students will take the position of Fig. 30, in which the backs of the hands are up.

No. 69.—*First Movements*—UP. At this command, the knit hands and the arms are stretched up as high as possible, as at A, in Fig. 30, and brought back to the commencing position four times; then four similar motions are made up and front at an angle of 45 degrees; and finally, eight motions from this position are made alternately in these two directions. *Rise on the toes with each upward motion.*

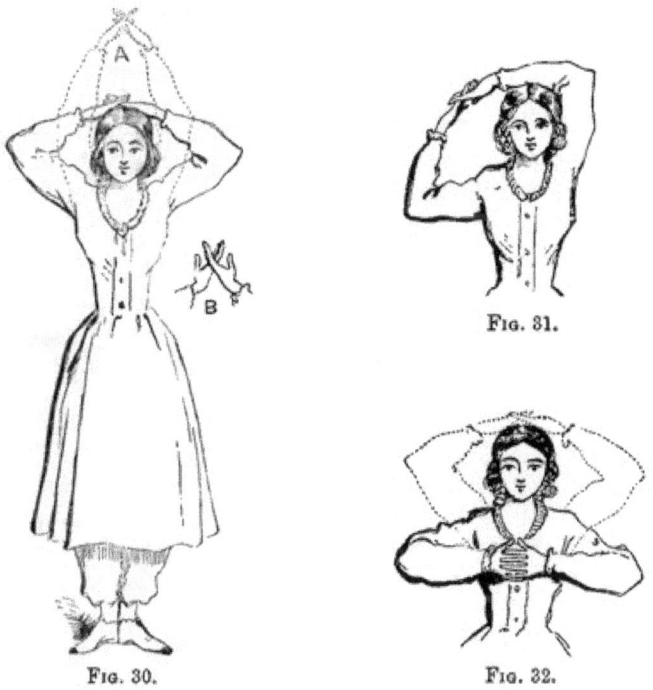

FIG. 30. FIG. 31. FIG. 32.

No. 70.—*Second Movements*—RIGHT. At this command, the hands and the arms will move to the right until the left elbow touches the head, as seen in Fig. 31, and recover the commencing position four times; when, at the command, LEFT, four corresponding motions will be made to the left; then, at the command, ALTERNATE, four motions from the fifth position will be made to the right and left alternately; and finally, at the command, BOTH, eight motions will be made the whole distance to the right and left, recovering the commencing position only on the eighth motion after the command, BOTH.

No. 71.—*Third Movements*—FRONT. The remaining commands are, BACK, ALTERNATE, BOTH. The number and order of the motions of the *third* class of movements from the fifth position are the same as the *second*, No. 70; but the motions are made from the head down to the front, as in Fig. 32, and behind, touching the back as low down as possible with the thumbs.

SECOND SERIES.

First Position.

No. 72.—The instructor will command: 1. *Elbow Exercise;* 2. *Second Series.* The remaining commands, the positions, the classes of movements, and the order, direction, and number of motions, are the same in the Second Series as in the First; with only the difference that the fingers are interlaced as at B, Fig. 30, thus bringing the backs of the hands *within*, and reversing the action of all of the muscles employed. *The positions of the backs of the hands, in all stages of execution of the movements of the First Series, must be reversed in the Second.*

Music.—When music is employed with Calisthenics or Gymnastics, the instructor will have the pieces, arranged for each general division, thoroughly tested, and use the music that is best adapted to the class of movements under consideration at the time. For example, the music on p. 55 is better adapted to the movements of Nos. 62 and 67, than that on p. 54: the music for Arm and Hand Exercise, commencing on p. 56, Part First, is better adapted to the movements of the First Position, p. 65; and Part Second, to the movements of the Second Position, p. 66.

IV.

ARM AND HAND EXERCISE.

FIRST SERIES.

First Position.

No. 73.—The instructor will command: 1. *Arm and Hand Exercise;* 2. *First Series;* 3. *First*—POSITION.

No. 74.—At the word, POSITION, the students will extend their arms directly front, and place the palms of the hands together, as in Fig. 33.

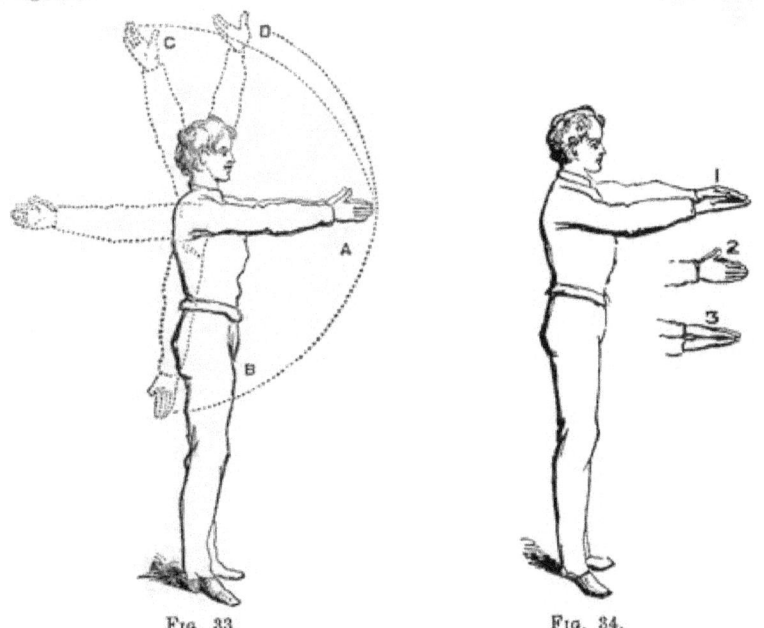

Fig. 33.　　　　　Fig. 34.

No. 75.—*First Movements*—RIGHT. At this command, the student will describe the line A B, Fig. 33, with the right hand, and recover the commencing position four times; at the command, LEFT, four corresponding motions from the position will be made with the left hand; at the command, ALTERNATE, four of these motions will be made from the position by alternation; and finally, at the command, BOTH, four of these motions will be made from the position with both hands simultaneously. Every time the commencing position is resumed, the palms will be struck together smartly, so as to mark the time.—Music for these exercises commences on p. 56.

No. 76.—*Second Movements*—RIGHT. The remaining commands, and the number and order of the movements, are the same as in No. 75; the motions being made directly back from the commencing position, as represented by the dotted arms at the rear in Fig. 33.

No. 77.—*Third Movements*—RIGHT. These movements, which correspond to those of No. 75, are made in the arcs A C and A D.

Second Position.

No. 78.—At the command, *Second*—POSITION, the arms are extended front, the palms are placed together, and the thumbs pointed to the right, as at 1, in Fig. 34.

No. 79.—*First Movements*—RIGHT; LEFT; RECIPROCATE. In executing these movements, the right palm strikes the left four drawn blows toward the breast, and then four similar ones in the opposite direction; the same number of corresponding blows is then given the right palm with the left; and, finally, one arm is thrust forward at the same time the other is drawn toward the breast, producing a seesaw or reciprocating motion, and the palms, when passing, are vigorously struck together until sixteen blows are given. The sixteen strokes produced by reciprocation are made with twice the rapidity of the preceding ones.—The *Second Movements* are executed with the hands held as at 2, in Fig. 34; the *Third*, as at 3. The number, order, direction, and kind of motions of each of the last two classes of movements, are the same as those of the first. These movements are valuable for the exercise of nearly all of the arm muscles, especially the flexors and the muscles of the fore-part of the chest.

Third Position.

No. 80.—At the command, *Third*—POSITION, which really involves four positions, the hands are held in line with the elbows, the right within the left and the thumbs pointed front, as represented at A, in Fig. 35.

No. 81.—*First Movements*—Right. At this command, the student will raise the right hand nearly to the chin, and bring it down, striking the palm of the left hand with the back of the right, four times; at the command, Left, he will strike the right hand with the left, in like manner, four times; and finally, at the command, Alternate, he will give eight blows alternately, first striking the left hand with the right. He will strike the hands together, on both odd and even numbers.—*Second Movements.* The second movements only differ from the first in being executed with the palms of the hands down, and the thumbs pointed toward the abdomen.

.No. 82.—*Third Movements*—Right. At this command, the student will first elevate the hands in line with, and about eight inches in front of the breast, the back of the right hand being held against the palm of the left and the thumbs pointed up, as represented at B in Fig. 35. He will then proceed to execute the movements, which only differ from the first class of movements of No. 81 in the direction of the motions, which is toward and from the breast. —*Fourth Movements.* These only differ from the *Third* in being executed with the palms to the front and the thumbs pointed down.

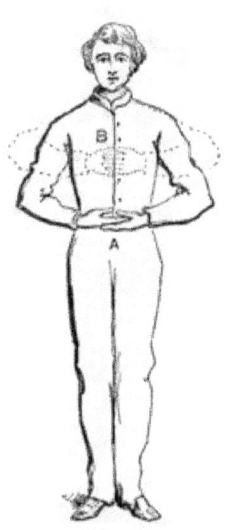

Fig. 35.

Fourth Position.

No. 83.—*Fourth*—Position. This varied position is taken in four places. On the word, Position, the arms are extended, and the palms are pressed together, as at A, Fig. 36, for the first place; and each remaining place is taken at the command, Change,—the second place being at B; the third, at C; and the fourth, in front at about the height of A, in Fig. 35, with the palms pressed together as at D, Fig. 36, the right thumb pointed toward the abdomen, and the left directly front.

No. 84.—*First Movements.* The first class of movements is executed by rubbing the palms vigorously together with a reciprocating or see-saw motion while rapidly counting eight *twice* at each

68   CALISTHENICS.

place named in No. 83.—The *Second Movements* are executed by rapidly striking the palms together eight times in each of the four places of the fourth position.

Fifth Position.

No. 85.—*Fifth*—Position. In this position, the arms are extended, *first* to the right in line with the chest, the thumbs being placed against the ends of the little fingers, with the ends of all the fingers in line with the thumbs, as in Fig. 37; *second*, the arms are

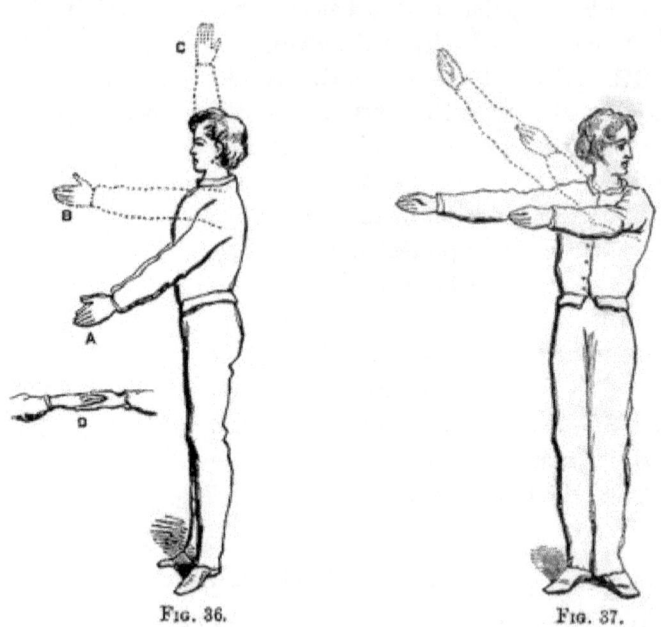

Fig. 36.   Fig. 37.

elevated on the same side, at an angle of 45 degrees, as represented by the dotted arms of Fig. 37; *third* and *fourth*, the arms are extended in two directions to the left, corresponding with those to the right; *fifth*, the arms are extended directly front in line with the shoulders; and *sixth*, the arms are extended front and up, at an angle of 45 degrees, corresponding to the position of the dotted arms of Fig. 37. When the arms are extended to the *right*, the face is turned to the *left*, and *vice versâ*. In extending the arms front, the head will be held erect, and the face front.

No. 86.—*First Movements*—RIGHT. The remaining commands are: UP; LEFT, UP; FRONT, UP; or the general command, *Change*, will answer for all of the commands but, RIGHT. The first and only class of movements is executed by extending the arms in the first four directions of No. 85, and simultaneously rubbing the ends of the thumbs against the ends of all of the fingers (*snapping the fingers*) *four* times in each direction; and finally, the arms are extended in the two directions front, and the fingers are snapped *eight* times in each of these positions.

SECOND SERIES.

First Position.

No. 87.—The instructor will command: 1. *Arm and Hand Exercise;* 2. *Second Series;* 3. *First*—POSITION.

No. 88.—At the third command, the student will take the first position, as in Fig. 38, in which the palms are up and the thumbs pointed back.

No. 89.—*First Movements.* The first class of movements is executed from the first position by tightly clinching the fingers, thus forming fists, on odd numbers, and stretching them out, as far as possible, on even numbers, four times, with the palms up; four times with the palms turned down; four times with the thumbs up; and four times with the thumbs down.

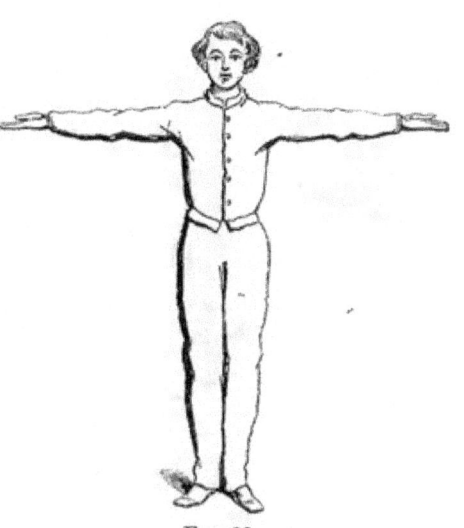

FIG. 38.

No. 90.—In all arm and hand exercises, when the arms are extended their full length, either sidewise or to the front, the palms will always have precedence, being held first *up* while a prescribed number of motions are being made, and then *down* during the same period; after which the thumbs are pointed up while the prescribed motions are being made, and then turned down for an equal period. The order and direction of these four modes of holding the hands are represented in Fig. 39.

No. 91.—*Second Movements.* The second class of movements from the position of Fig. 38, will be executed by first turning the arms so that the thumbs point front with the palms down on odd numbers, and recovering the commencing position on even ones four times; second, with the arms still extended sidewise, and the hands held so that the thumbs point up as at 3 in Fig. 39, turn the arms so that the thumbs shall describe arcs front and point down, the palms being back, four times; and finally, with the palms up, turn the arms and hands completely over, and recover the commencing position eight times. In describing the last eight motions from the commencing position, the arms will be so turned that the palms shall be up on both odd and even numbers, differing only from Fig. 40 at the termination of the motion from the commencing position, in having the arms extended sidewise.

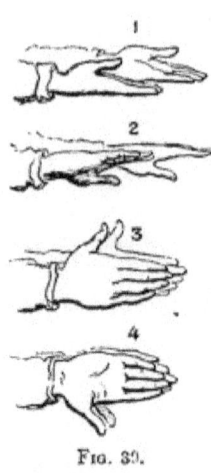

Fig. 39.

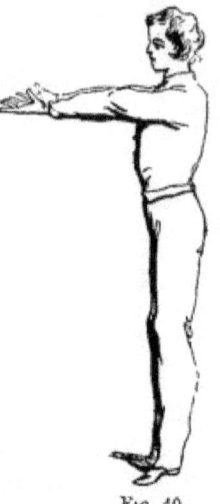

Fig. 40.

No. 92.—*Third Movements*—Reciprocate. At this command, *from the position of Fig.* 38, the trunk vibrates from side to side, bending as much as possible, *with the legs kept straight,* first to the right and then to the left, *eight* times for each of the four modes of holding the hands described in No. 90. On the *thirty-second* motion the commencing position is resumed. When the trunk bends to the right, the right arm is depressed and the left one elevated; and when the trunk bends to the left, the left arm is depressed and the right one elevated, thus describing the motion of Fig. 41. This class of movements, with some others of the Series, is both an Arm and Hand, and a Trunk exercise. Indeed, it brings in play, very pleasantly and effectively, nearly all the muscles of the body. Let it be executed frequently.

Second Position.

No. 93.—At the command, *Second*—POSITION, the student will take the position of Fig. 42, in which the arms are extended horizontally front, in line with the shoulders, with the palms up.

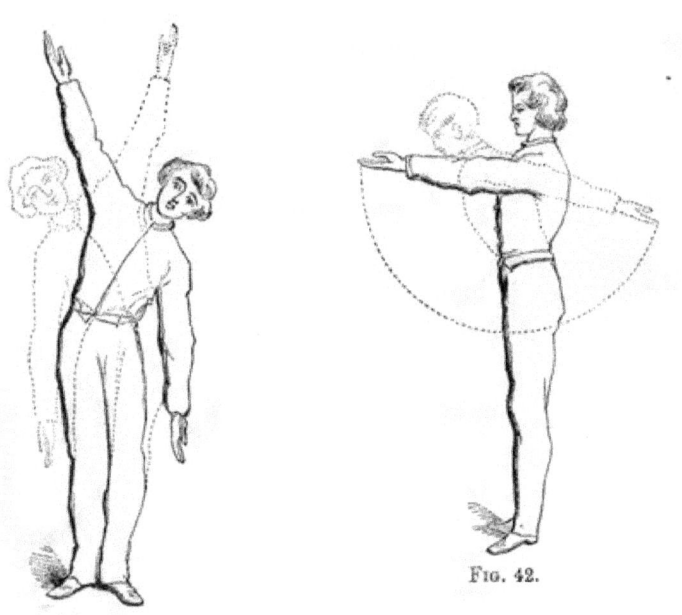

Fig. 41.   Fig. 42.

No. 94.—*First Movements.*[1] This class of movements corresponds to that of No. 89.—*Second Movements.* The second class of movements of this position is executed by turning the palms to the *second* direction of Fig. 39, and back to the *first*, four times; then to the *fourth*, and back to the *third*, four times; and, finally, the arms are turned completely over from the position of Fig. 42 to that of Fig. 40, and back again, eight times.

---

[1] **Effects of Movements.**—The four classes of movements described in Nos. 89, 91, and 94, bring into play the rotatory muscles of the arm and hand, and the finger muscles. They promote a free action of the joints of the arm, the wrist, and the fingers, and are, besides, useful against paralyzation of the above-mentioned muscles, and contractions of the wrist and finger-joints. Students will frequently execute these movements.

No. 95.—*Third Movements (Rocking Exercise).*[1] These movements are executed by throwing the arms forcibly backward and forward sixteen times; that is, four times for each of the four directions of the hands in Fig. 39. As the arms and hands are recovering the commencing position for the fourth time, the command, CHANGE, is given, and the direction of the palms, or thumbs, is changed and the movements continued. The trunk must not remain stiff, but rather yielding upon the hip joints in such a manner that, acting as a balance, it is now bent a little forward, now a little backward, as represented by the dotted part of Fig. 42. The whole movement is thereby rendered easier, and the effect more universal.

Third Position.

No. 96.—At the command, *Third*—POSITION, the student will take the position of Fig. 43, in which the right palm is placed upon the back of the left hand, the head is drawn back, the chin elevated, the breast projected, and the back hollowed.

No. 97.—*First Movements.* The first and only class of movements from this position is executed by first bending the trunk to the left, and describing two arcs simultaneously with the hands out and back, at an angle of 45 degrees, and recovering the commencing position, four times (see Fig. 43), as though one were swimming partially on the left side; then the trunk is bent in like manner to the right, and four corresponding double motions are simultaneously executed from the position, as though one were swimming partially on the right side;

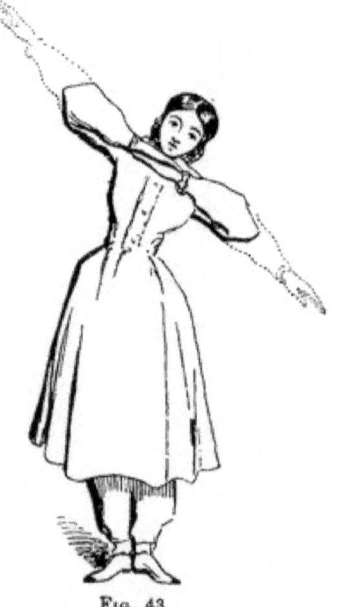

FIG. 43.

---

[1] **Third Movements.**—In executing the movements of Nos. 92 and 95, not only the respective arm and shoulder muscles, but most of those of the abdomen, the sides, and the back, are set in a sort of *rocking motion*. The immediate effect of this motion is an agreeable feeling; and although the motion itself is somewhat violent, its influence is, on the

and, finally, standing erect, with the elbows in line with the shoulders, eight outward motions are made with both arms simultaneously, as though a swimmer were striking out directly in front. On every outward movement from the commencing position, the student rises on the toes, and stretches the whole body upward and forward.

THIRD SERIES.

First Position.

No. 98.—The instructor commands: 1. *Arm and Hand Exercise;* 2. *Third Series;* 3. *First*—POSITION.

No. 99.—At the third command, the student will take the position of Fig. 44, with the arms extended horizontally, and the palms up, as at A and C.

No. 100.——*First Movements*—RIGHT. At this command, the right arm will describe the arc A B and recover the commencing position four times; then, at the command, LEFT, the left arm will describe the arc C D, and recover the commencing position four times; then, at the command, ALTERNATE, four corresponding downward motions will be made with

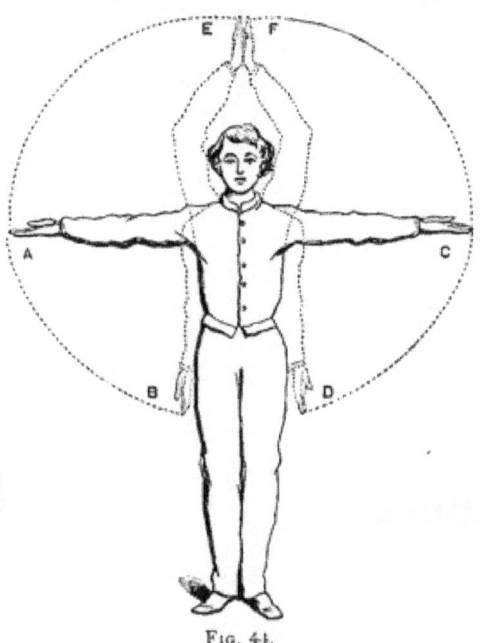

FIG. 44.

whole, a mild one. It forms, first, a pretty good quota of the whole amount of exercise required, and is a powerful promoter of the circulation of the blood. It is also of essential service in cases of paralyzation of the muscles of the arm, back, and abdomen, as well as sluggishness and interruption of the functions of the abdomen in general, and is recommended on account of its mild working in special cases, and particularly as a rest during the execution of a series of calisthenic exercises. Althe arms alternately; and, finally, at the command, BOTH, the arcs A B and C D will be described, and the commencing position regained four times with both arms simultaneously.

No. 101.—*Second Movements*—RIGHT. The remaining commands, and the number and order of the motions, are the same as those of No. 100; but this class of movements is executed in the arcs A E and C F. In raising the arms separately, they are to be carried up only to a vertical position; but when both arms are raised simultaneously, the palms are vigorously brought together over the head, as represented in Fig. 44.

No. 102.—*Third Movements.*[1] The only remaining command of this class of movements, CHANGE, is employed three times. First, the right arm will describe the arc A B, and the left C F, and recover the commencing position four times simultaneously; then the right arm will describe the arc A E, and the left C D, and recover the commencing position four times in like manner; then the right arm will describe the arc A B at the same time the left is describing C F, when the right arm will describe the entire arc B A E, and the left F C D, simultaneously, only stopping at the commencing position, A and C, after the right hand has been at B and the left at F four times; and, finally, both arms will pass up to E and F, and then describe simultaneously the complete arcs E A B and F C D, and immediately regain the position of the dotted arms at E F, only stopping at the commencing position, A and C, on the fourth downward motion.

Second Position.

No. 103.—At the command, *Second—*POSITION, the students will take the position of Fig. 42, which only differs from the position

---

though the movement is not what may be called heating (in spite of the impulse given to the blood), yet it may be advantageously used for warming the trunk, arms, and hands. It has a favorable effect as a stimulant at those times of bodily and mental lassitude which now and then arrive, in consequence sometimes of a change in the weather or of the season, or of a disarranged state of the nervous system of the abdomen, and which are not to be otherwise explained. If thought necessary, these classes of movements may be executed several times.

[1] **The movements** of this position bring into play the allotment or raising muscles of the arm, and the side-neck muscles, enlarge the sides of the chest and the space between the lower ribs, and promote healthy respiration.

of No. 99 in having the arms extended directly *front*, in line with the shoulders

No. 104.—The three classes of movements from this position have the same number and order of motions, and the same commands, as Nos. 100, 101, and 102, respectively; but they are executed in front of the body instead of to the sides.

Third Position.

No. 105.—At the command, *Third*—Position, the student will take the position of Fig. 45, in which the arms and hands are as at A A.

No. 106.——*First Movements.*——These movements are executed from the sides by bending both elbows simultaneously, and drawing the forearms in on odd numbers and straightening the arms on even ones, first from A A to B B, Fig. 45; from B B to C C; from C C to D D; from D D to E E; and then back, by reversing the order of the motions. These motions will be made in regular order from A A to E E and back,

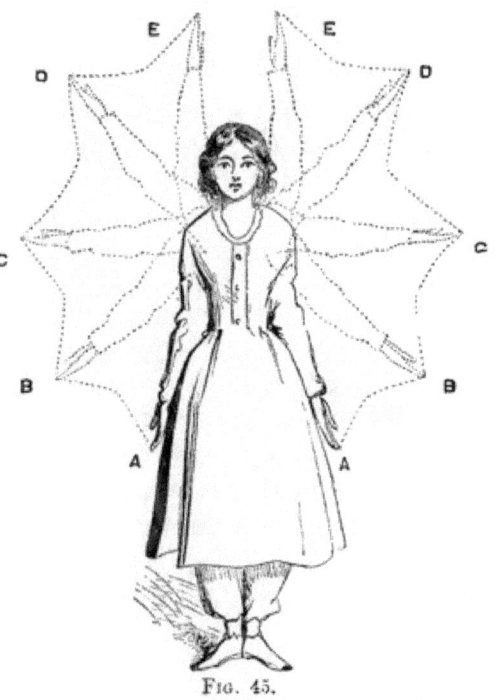

Fig. 45.

twice with the palms out at the sides and the thumbs back; and twice with the backs of the hands out and the thumbs pointed front.

No. 107.—*Second Movements.* The second class of movements is made in front, as represented by Fig. 46. In its execution, the elbows are bent and the arms thrust simultaneously forward, in such a manner as to form the irregular line B C D E F. When counting is employed, the arms will be at A C on *two;* at A D, on *four;* at A E, on *six;* and at A F, on *eight;* when the direction of the motions is reversed, and the arms resume the position A B on the second *eight.* These motions are made in front from B to F, and back from F to B, once with the palms held front and up; once with the backs of the hands front and up; once with the thumbs pointed front and up; and once with the thumbs pointed back and down, see Fig. 39.

FOURTH SERIES.

First Position.

No. 108.—The instructor commands: 1. *Arm and Hand Exercise;* 2. *Fourth Series;* 3. *First*—POSITION.

No. 109.—At the last command, the student will take the position of Fig. 47.

No. 110.—*First Movements (Chopping).* The first and only class of movements from this position is executed by first making the motion represented by the dotted part of Fig. 47, and recovering the commencing position eight times; and then taking the position on the left side, with the left hand higher than the right, like a left-handed chopper, and making eight corresponding downward motions inclining to the right. The accent will be placed upon the downward motions.

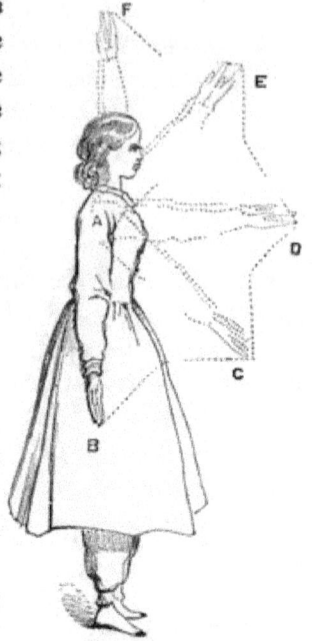

Fig. 46.

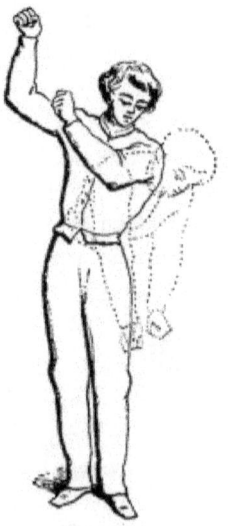

Fig. 47.

Second Position.

No. 111.—At the command, *Second*—POSITION, the student will take the position of Fig. 48.

No. 112.—The movements of this position correspond to those of No. 110; but the eight motions from the right side are made by throwing the arms up, as represented by the dotted part of Fig. 48. Eight corresponding upward motions are made from the left side, the motions to recover the commencing position being unaccented. These are the motions of a chopper, who is chopping into a tree as high as possible above his head.

Third Position.

No. 113.—At the command, *Third— Position (Sawing)*, the student will take the position of Fig. 49, in which the body is bent slightly forward, inclining to the right, and principally supported on the right foot; the arms are bent at the elbows, and the left fist is held higher than the right, as though one were holding a buck-saw in position to give a downward stroke.

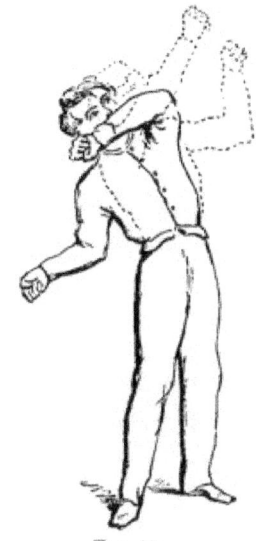

Fig. 48.

No. 114.—*First Movements*—Down. At this command, the arms are thrust down slightly inclining front, as represented by the dotted arms of Fig. 49, and instantly brought back to the commencing position sixteen times; when, at the command, Change, the body is inclined to the left, its weight being principally thrown on the left foot, the position of the hands is reversed, and sixteen corresponding downward motions are made to the left. The motions to recover the commencing position are made by bending the elbows as in sawing firewood. *The air will be audibly expired on each downward motion, producing the sound represented by the combination* sh, *and inspired on each upward motion, taking care to have the lungs fully inflated each time the commencing*

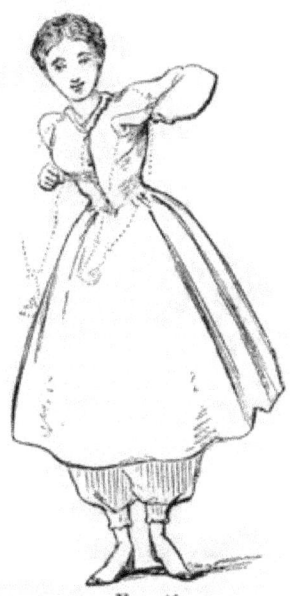

Fig. 49.

4*

position is regained. These movements contribute much to the amount of necessary universal action, and exercise the chest, and nearly all the muscles of the arm, shoulder, and back.

Fourth Position.

No. 115.—*Fourth*—POSITION (*Mowing*). At this command, the student, advancing the right leg and foot, and extending the arms to the right, will take the position of Fig. 50, in which the body is bent forward a little, to give free action to the arms. This is the position of one who is mowing grass on level ground. This position varies twice during the execution of the movements: first, to that of Fig. 51, in which the body is upright and the arms are stretched directly to the right, as though one standing in a ditch were mowing in line with the breast; and, second, the body is bent a little back, and the arms held to the right, inclining up, as though one mowing on a side-hill were reaching higher than his head, as in Fig. 52.

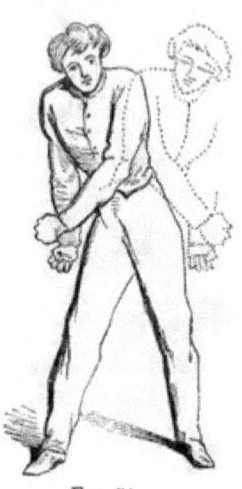

FIG. 50.

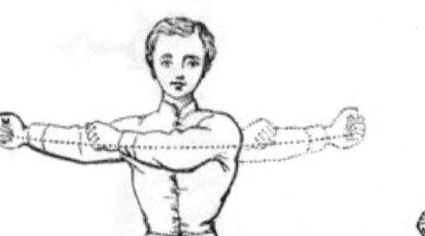

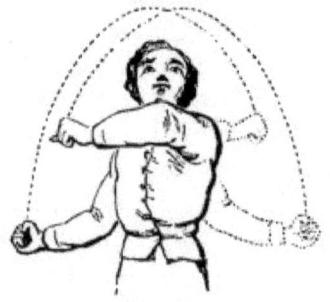

FIG. 51.   FIG. 52.

No. 116.—*First Movements.*[1] In describing the first and only class of movements from the Fourth Position, the feet remain immov-

---

[1] These movements cause a lively activity, not only of the muscles of the shoulders and the allotment mus- cles of the arms, but also a sort of see-saw stretching of all the muscles of the trunk, leg, and foot. They

able, and the arms describe semicircles alternately to the left, and then back to the right. One should imagine one's self mowing both *left* and *right*, in which motion a certain *force* is exerted in the act of swinging. The accent must be laid equally upon the movement to the left and that to the right. The students will describe eight semicircles of Fig. 50; eight, of Fig. 51; and sixteen, of Fig. 52. These semicircles are made with both arms simultaneously. This class of movements should be repeated before passing to the next Series.

FIFTH SERIES.

First Position.

No. 117.—The instructor will command: 1. *Arm and Hand Exercise;* 2. *Fifth Series;* 3. *First*—POSITION.

No. 118.—At the third command, the students will take the position of Fig. 53, in which the forearms are placed upon the hips, with the fists extended just in front of the waist, and their backs out to the sides.

No. 119.—*First Movements.* The first class of movements is executed by first describing, with both hands simultaneously, sixteen outward circles, and then sixteen inward ones, as represented by the dotted circles of Fig. 53.

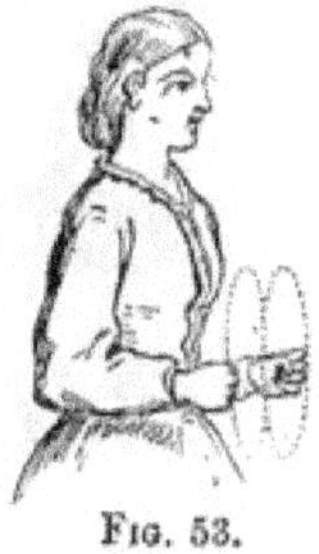

No. 120.—*Second Movements.* This class of movements only differs from No. 119 in being executed with the *elbows* upon the *hips*, thus describing larger circles, as represented in Fig. 54.

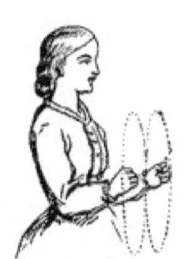

FIG. 53.

FIG. 54.

Second Position.

No. 121.—At the command, *Second*—POSITION, the student will take the position of Fig. 55, in which the right hand is held about five inches above the left, with both palms up and the thumbs pointed front.

---

have, therefore, an invigorating influence upon the limb-moving muscles of the whole body, and are of great service in cases of a general muscular weakness, and of paralyzation of the spinal marrow.

80 CALISTHENICS.

No. 122.—*First Movements.* The movements are executed by moving the hands rapidly around each other in circles, as in Fig. 55, describing sixteen *inward* circles (eight with each hand) and sixteen *outward* ones, with the palms up; and then, at the command, CHANGE, without changing the relative position of the hands, the palms are turned down and the thumbs pointed toward the abdomen, when sixteen additional *inward* and sixteen *outward* circles are described. At the *second* command, CHANGE, the right hand is held above the left, with the palms in and the thumbs pointed up; at the *third*, without changing the relative position of the hands, the palms are turned front and the thumbs pointed down. Sixteen *inward* and sixteen *outward* circles are executed with the thumbs pointed up, and the same number with the thumbs pointed down.

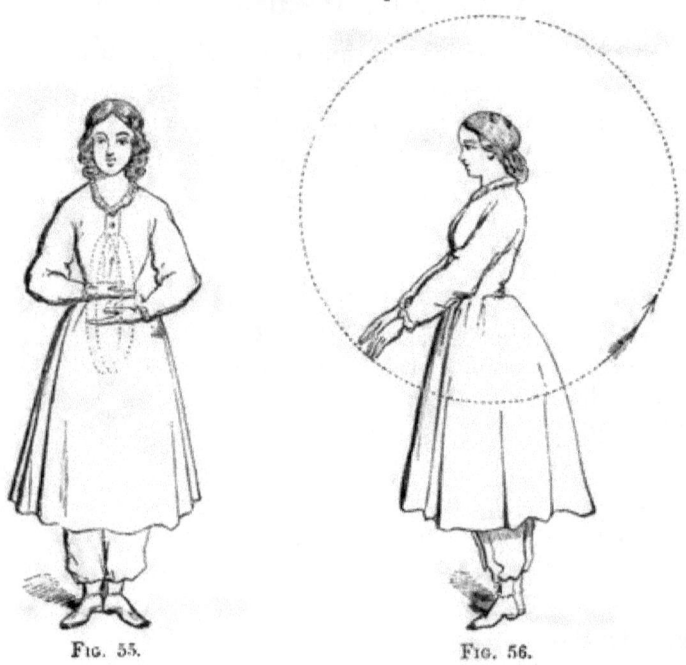

FIG. 55.   FIG. 56.

Third Position.

No. 123.—At the command, *Third*—POSITION, the position taken is that of Fig. 56, in which the arms and the backs of the hands are extended front at an angle of 45 degrees.

No. 124.—*First Movements*—RIGHT. At this command, the

right arm will describe eight as large side circles as possible, in a backward direction, as indicated by the arrow in Fig. 56; then, at the command, LEFT, the left arm will describe eight corresponding circles; then, at the command, ALTERNATE, eight corresponding circles will be described with the arms alternately, the left arm commencing a circle just before the right arm has regained its commencing position, thus rendering the circle continuous; and, finally, at the command, BOTH, eight corresponding circles will be described with both arms simultaneously. *All side and head circles will be described in the direction of the palms,* the students standing with the feet in the military position, and bringing the arms close to the head while executing the movements.

Fourth Position.

No. 125.—At the command, *Fourth*—POSITION, the student will take the position of Fig. 57. The number, order, and kind of motions[1] from this position are the same as those of No. 124; but the circles are described in the direction indicated by the arrow in Fig. 57.

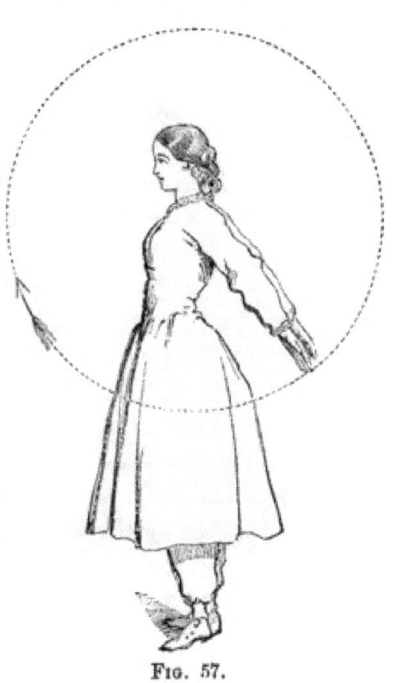

FIG. 57.

Fifth Position.

No. 126.—At the command, *Fifth*—POSITION, the student will take the position of Fig. 58, in which the elbows are extended to the sides, and the hands are held over the head with the palms front.

---

[1] **The movements** of Nos. 124 and 125 cause a freedom of action of the shoulders, promote respiration, and enlarge the framework of the chest. They may be improved upon by inflating the lungs with a full inspiration, and then holding the breath while these circular motions are made as described above. This is one of the very best methods of enlarging the capacity of the air-cells of the lungs.

No. 127.—*First Movements*—RIGHT. These movements are executed by describing circles over the head in the direction of the palms: First, eight circles are described with the right arm; then, eight with the left; and finally, sixteen circles are described with both arms simultaneously, as represented in Fig. 58. A circle is completed on every number counted.

No. 128.——*Second Movements*—RIGHT. In executing these movements, the backs of the hands are held front, with the thumbs up. The number of circles, and the order of their execution, are the same as in No. 127; but they are described in an opposite direction. These movements cause a freedom of the action of the shoulders, of the elbows, and of the wrists, and bring in play nearly all the muscles of the trunk. They may be rendered more interesting by occasionally executing them with a handkerchief in the hand, the time being marked by repeatedly shouting the word HURRAH (hoo rah'), as in giving hearty cheers. In this event, the trunk will first bend to the left, and the left arm will

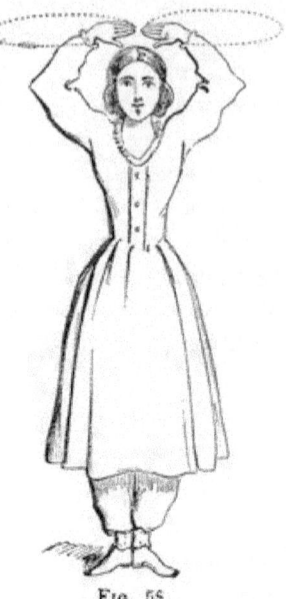

FIG. 58.

hang in its usual position by the side, while the right arm describes eight as large circles as possible with the handkerchief over the head; then the left arm will describe eight corresponding circles, the right arm being suspended by the side, and the trunk bent to the right. In shouting HURRAH, the first syllable will be uttered with twice the rapidity of the second. A circle will be described every time the first syllable is uttered, and then the arm will remain motionless long enough to utter the second syllable and to thoroughly inflate the lungs.

HEAD AND NECK EXERCISE.

H. B. DODWORTH.

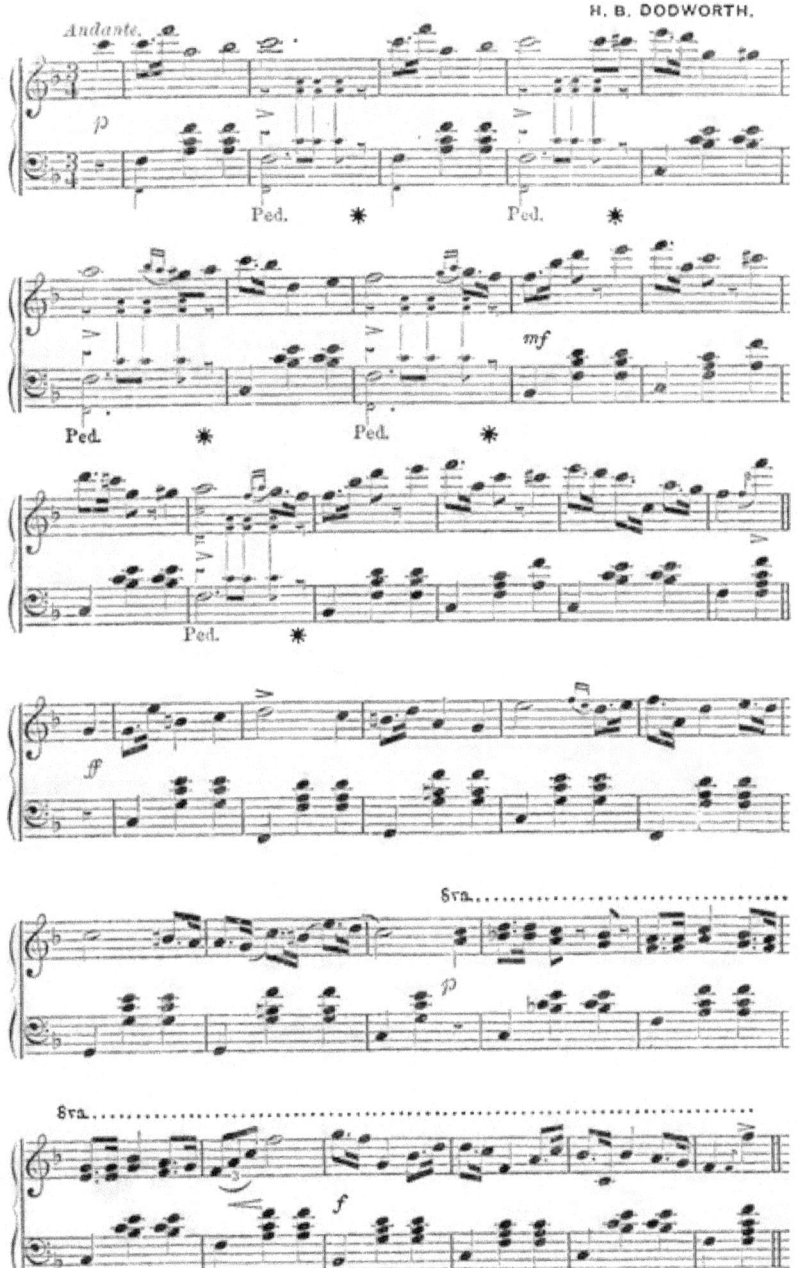

TRUNK AND WAIST EXERCISE.

J. LABITZKY.

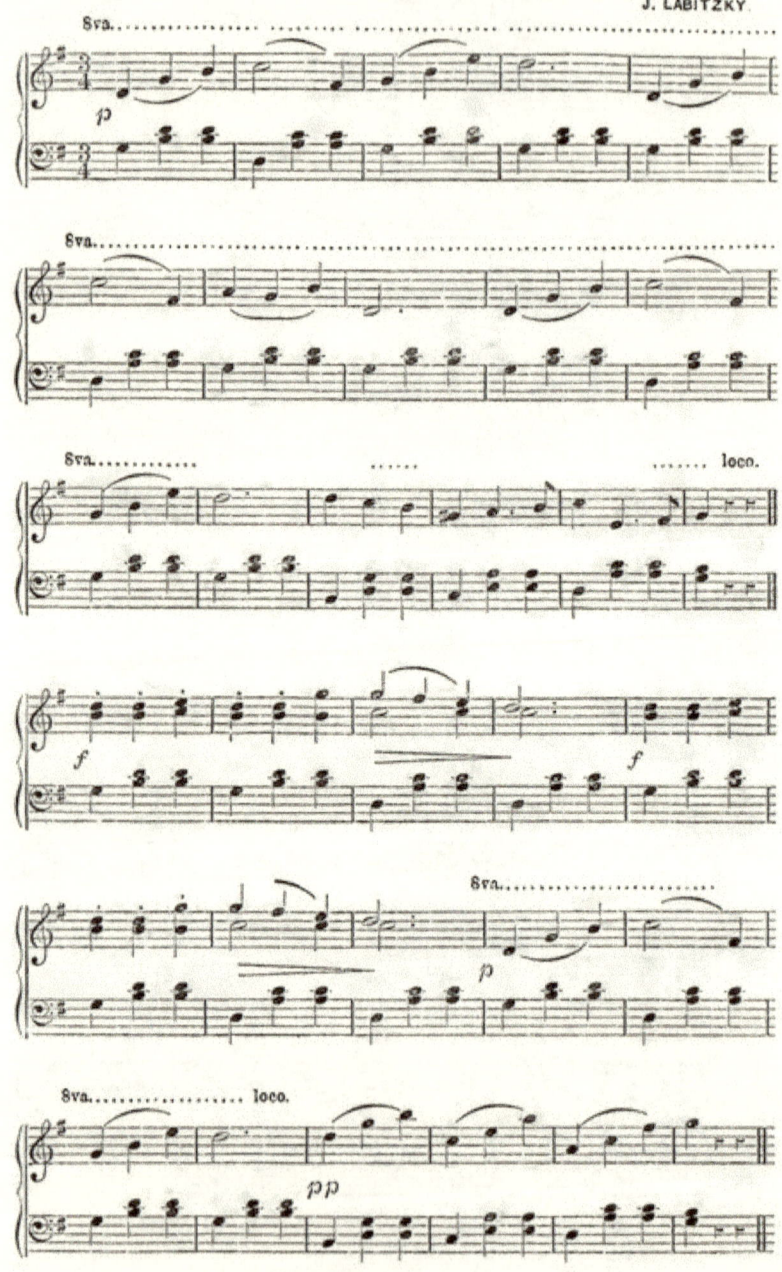

KNEE EXERCISE.

PART FIRST.

Andante.   J. LABITZKY.

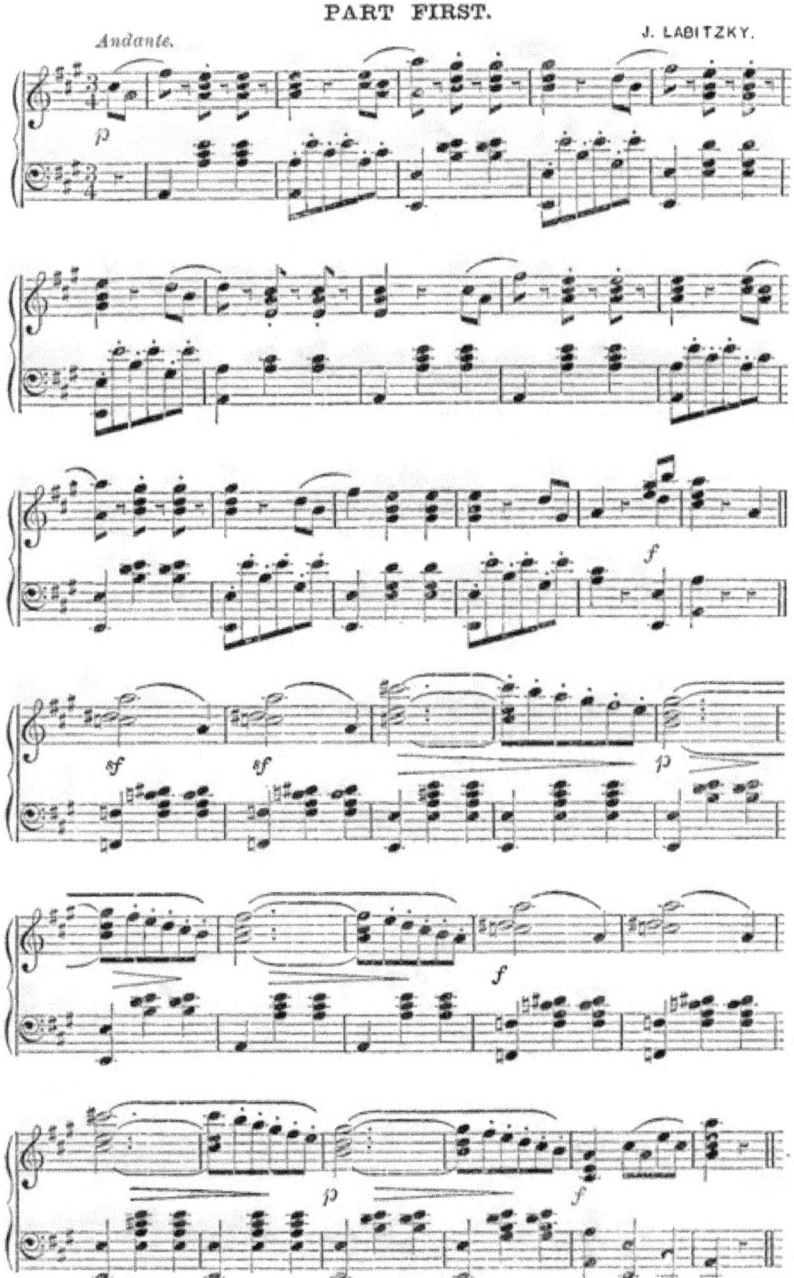

CALISTHENICS.

PART SECOND.

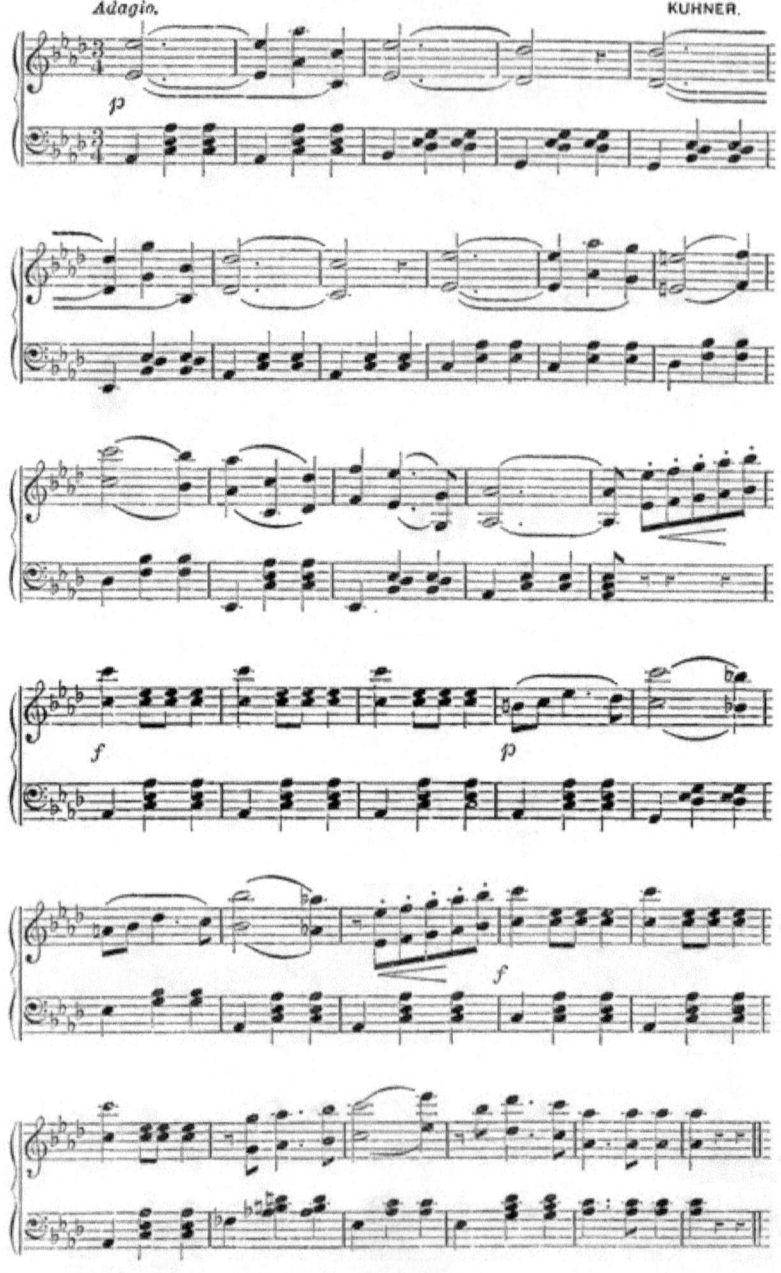

V.

HEAD AND NECK EXERCISE.

FIRST SERIES.

First Position.

No. 129.—The instructor will command: 1. *Head and Neck Exercise;* 2. *First Series;* 3. *First*—Position.

No. 130.—On the second word of the third command, the student will take the position from the *habitual* or *military* one, p. 10, by simply placing the hands back of and upon the hips, *with the thumbs front*, as represented in Fig. 59, the head being held vertical. The elbows will be forced down and back as far as possible. This is the position of the arms and hands for all the movements of the Series.

No. 131.—*First Movements*—Right. At this command, the head will bend down to the right, as represented by the dotted head of Fig. 60, and regain the commencing position four times; then, at the command, Left, four corresponding motions from the position will be made to the left; then, at the command, Alternate, four of these motions will be made alternately, first to the *right* and back to the commencing position, and then to the *left*; and finally, at the command, Both, eight motions will be made completely over from side to side, the first motion commencing from, and the eighth terminating at, the commencing position. All the movements of the head and neck are to be done in slow time. They comprise *flexions, turnings,* and *extensions*. In executing the flexions of this class of movements, the head is exactly bent to the side designated, without

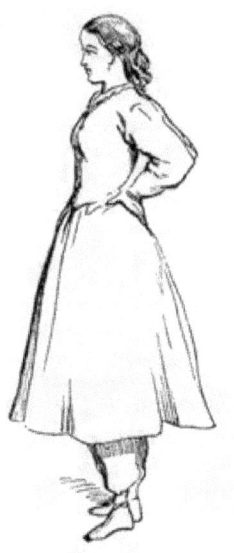

Fig. 59.

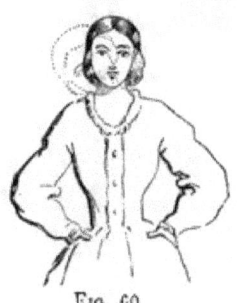

Fig. 60.

twisting the face or shoulders, and with no raising of the opposite shoulder, nor sinking down of the shoulder on the same side.

No. 132.—*Second Movements.* The commands of execution are: 1. FRONT; 2. BACK; 3. ALTERNATE; 4. BOTH. In the commencing position the head is vertical. The movements are executed directly front and back, as represented in Fig. 61. The number of motions, and the order in which they are made, are the same as in No. 131.

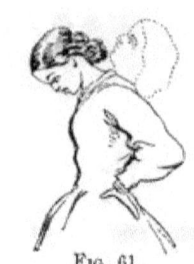

FIG. 61.

No. 133.—*Third Movements*—RIGHT. These movements are executed by first turning the head horizontally to the right side, without the least flexion, so as to bring the inner corner of the left eye in line with the eyes of students in, or supposed to be in, the same rank, as in Fig. 62, and regaining the commencing position four times; then four corresponding motions from the commencing position will be made to the left; then four of these motions will be made alternately, first to the *right* and back to the commencing position, and then to the *left;* and finally, eight motions will be made from side to side, describing one half of a circle with the head at each turning, only the first motion commencing from, and the eighth terminating at, the commencing position.

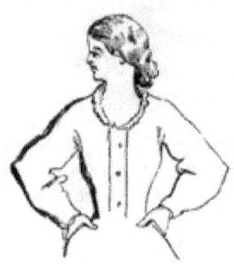

FIG. 62.

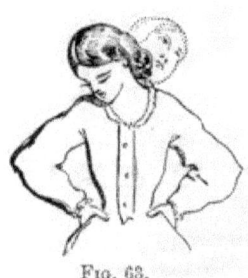

FIG. 63.

Second Position.

No. 134.—At the command, *Second*—POSITION, the neck will be bent first to the right, and the head lowered as far as possible, as represented by the dotted head of Fig. 60.

No. 135.—*First Movements.* These movements are executed by first describing four circles with the head and neck from the right shoulder, the head advancing to the front before passing over the

HEAD AND NECK EXERCISE. 89

left shoulder, as represented in Fig. 63; then four circles are described from the right shoulder, the head being carried to the rear before passing over the left shoulder; then the position is taken over the left shoulder, and four circles are described by moving the head to the rear before it passes over the right shoulder; and finally, four circles are described from the left shoulder by advancing the head to the front before it passes over the right shoulder. The circumference of the circle will be as great as the articulation of the neck renders possible. Students will first employ the third variety of counting, p. 40, in connection with these movements. The chin passes over a shoulder on each accented number. These movements set all the muscles of the neck in motion, and render their action freer. They are a valuable remedy against nervous giddiness and stiffness of the neck.

SECOND SERIES.

First Position.

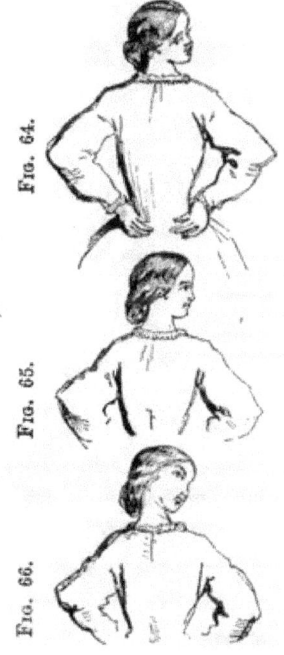

No. 136.—The instructor commands: 1. *Head and Neck Exercise;* 2. *Second Series;* 3. *First*—Position. At the last command, the students will take the position of Fig. 59.

No. 137.—*First Movements*—Right. At this command, the head is turned over the right shoulder, and the neck is stretched, *with a downward flexion*, as if one were trying to look at the heels, as in Fig. 64. As soon as the neck has been stretched *as far as possible*, the head is turned front and raised into the vertical position. This motion from the commencing position is described four times to the right; then, at the command, Left, a corresponding motion is described four times to the left; then, at the command, Alternate, four of these motions are made alternately, first to the right; and finally, at the command, Both, eight double motions are made from side to side, the first commencing from, and the eighth ending at, the commencing position. *All the movements of this Series are executed in very slow time.*

No. 138.—*Second Movements*—RIGHT. The remaining commands, and the number and order of the motions, are the same as in No. 137. In executing the movements, the head, held vertical, is *stretched over the shoulders as far as possible*, as though one were trying, without moving the feet or the trunk, to look at an object in line with the head directly in the rear, as represented in Fig. 65.

No. 139.—*Third Movements*—RIGHT. The remaining commands, and the number and order of these movements, are the same as in No. 137; but the motions are made by stretching the neck with an *upward* flexion of the head, as though one were trying to look at a mark on the ceiling directly back of, and in line with, the opposite shoulder, as in Fig. 66.

VI.

TRUNK AND WAIST EXERCISE.

FIRST SERIES.

First Position.

No. 140.—The instructor will command: 1. *Trunk and Waist Exercise;* 2. *First Series;* 3. *First*—POSITION.

No. 141.—At the last command, the student will take the position of the dotted part of Fig. 67, or of No. 130.

No. 142.—*First Movements*—RIGHT. The remaining commands are: 1. LEFT; 2. ALTERNATE; 3. BOTH. The movements are executed with the legs unbent and their muscles rigid. The trunk will first bend to the right *as far as possible*, as in Fig. 67, and recover the vertical position four times; then four corresponding motions will be made to the left; then four motions will be made to the sides alternately; and finally, eight motions will be made from side to

TRUNK AND WAIST EXERCISE. 91

side, the first commencing from, and the eighth terminating at, the commencing position. *All the movements are made energetically, but in slow time.*—Music for these exercises on p. 84.

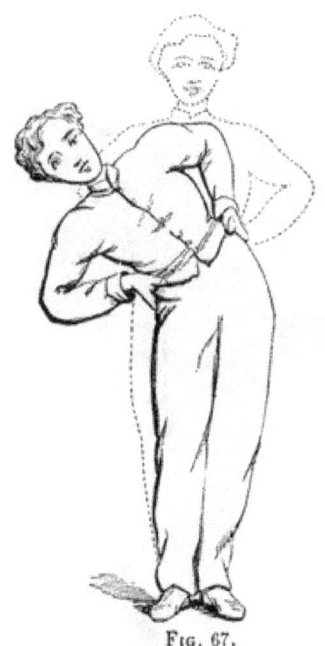

Fig. 67.

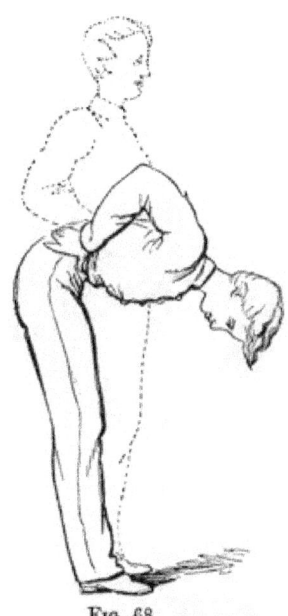

Fig. 68.

No. 143.—*Second Movements.* The commands of execution are: 1. Front; 2. Back; 3. Alternate; 4. Both. The number and order of these movements are the same as in No. 142; but the body is bent forward and backward instead of sidewise. When making the forward motions, *the legs and the spine are kept straight,* the bending taking place only at the hips, as in Fig. 68. The backward motions are usually made with the legs straight; but students will occasionally be required to bend backward as far as possible, as in Fig. 69.

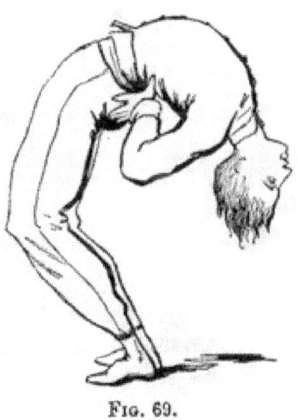

Fig. 69.

No. 144.—*Third Movements*—Right. The remaining commands, and the number and order of the motions, are the same as in

No. 142; but, in describing the movements, the trunk maintains its upright position, and turns on its axis the same distance on each side, the legs and feet being immovable, and the back well stretched, as in Fig. 70. The trunk turns to the *right* side only far enough to bring the inner corner of the left eye in line with the eyes of students in, or supposed to be in, the same rank, and the same distance to the *left*.

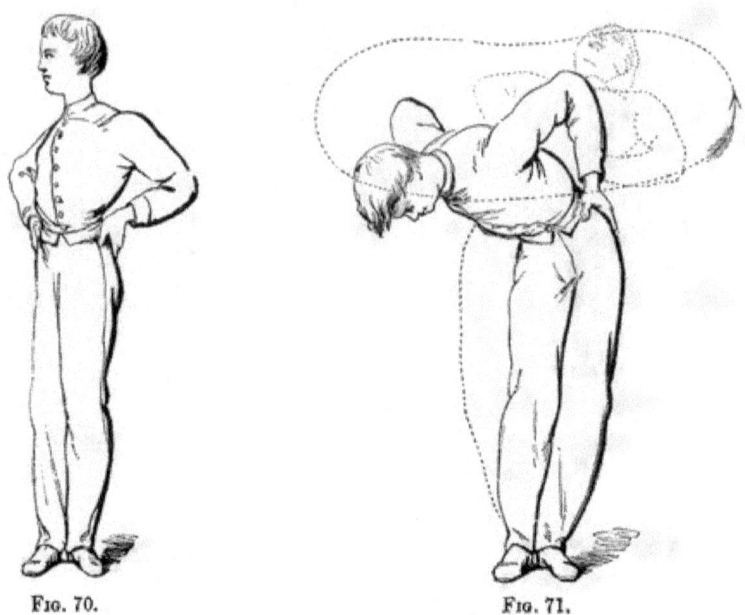

Fig. 70.   Fig. 71.

Second Position.

No. 145.—*Second*—Position. At this command, the body is bent sidewise, first to the right, as in Fig. 67, the legs remaining straight

No. 146.—*First Movements*. In executing these movements, the trunk, turning on the hips, advancing front from the right, as in Fig. 71, first describes four circles in the direction indicated by the arrow; then four circles are described in a contrary direction; then, with the position taken on the left side (the trunk bent to the left as far as possible), four circles will be described in the direction indicated by the arrow in Fig. 71; and finally, four circles will be described from the left in a contrary direction. The proper and equal exercise of the muscles of the trunk has a more direct and favorable influence on the health than that of any other member. These movements bring into play and strengthen all the muscles lying about the hips. They also give a sort of see-saw, alternate motion to the abdominal muscles. This motion gives a universal impulse to the digestive organs, and is therefore recommended in cases of sluggishness, and the many evils consequent thereupon. In cases of nervous giddiness, these movements must at first be practiced sitting.

SECOND SERIES.

First Position.

No. 147.—The instructor commands: 1. *Trunk and Waist Exercise;* 2. *Second Series;* 3. *First*—Position.

No. 148.—At the third command, the student will take the position of Fig. 59, which is the commencing position of the three classes of movements of this Series.

No. 149.—*First Movements*—Right. At this command, with the feet immovable, the trunk is turned over the right hip, and stretched, *with a downward flexion,* as in Fig. 72, sufficiently to enable the student to see the heels of those at the left in, or supposed to be in, the same rank, and then the commencing position is resumed. This movement is described four times to the right; then, at the command, Left, a corresponding movement is described four times to the left; then, at the command, Alternate, four of these movements are made from the commencing position alternately, first to the right; and finally, at the command, Both, eight combined movements are made, first describing a movement from the commencing position to the right, and then completely round and over to the left, only pausing at the commencing position on the eighth motion.

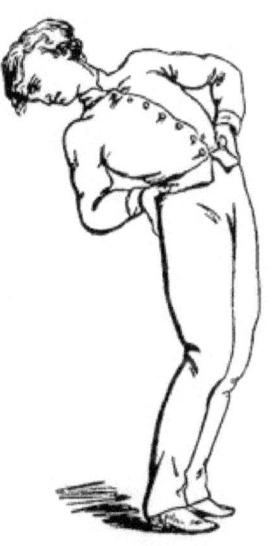

Fig. 72.

No. 150.—*Second Movements*—RIGHT. The remaining commands, and the number and order of the motions, are the same as in No. 149; but, in executing the movements, *the trunk, held vertical, is stretched over the hips as far as possible,* as though one, with his feet immovable, were trying to turn his back completely in front, see Fig. 73.

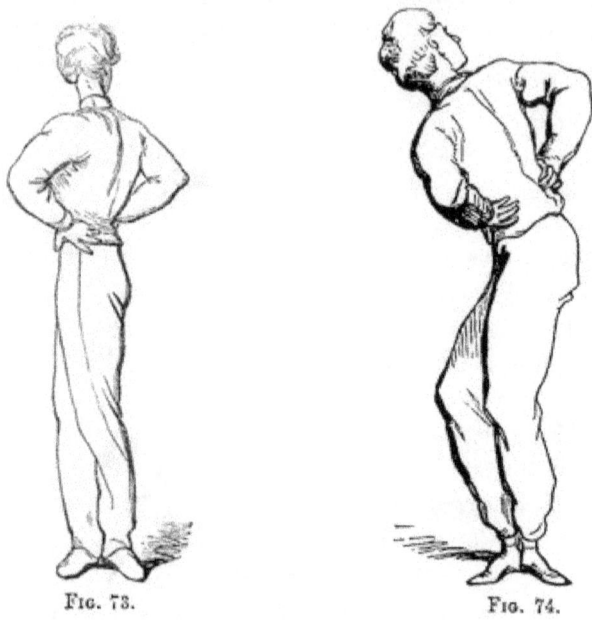

FIG. 73.   FIG. 74.

No. 151.—*Third Movements*—RIGHT. The remaining commands, and the number and order of this class of movements, are the same as No. 149; but the trunk, in describing the motions, is stretched with an *upward* flexion, as in Fig. 74.

No. 152.—While the three classes of movements immediately preceding, form a splendid Series of Trunk and Waist Exercises, they are much more than this: they embrace, in combination, energetic and invigorating exercise for the head and neck, trunk and waist, knee, and leg and foot, bringing into play nearly all the muscles of the body.

VII.

KNEE EXERCISE.

FIRST SERIES.

First Position.

No. 153.—The instructor will command: 1. *Knee Exercise;* 2. *First Series;*[1] 3. *First*—POSITION.

No. 154.—At the third command, the student will take the position by grasping the hips with the hands, turning the left foot so that it points directly front, and placing the right heel behind the left in such a manner that the feet form a right angle in front, as represented in Fig. 75. There are *nine* positions of the feet for the three classes of movements of the First Position. In the *first*, Fig. 76, the right heel is placed behind the left, forming a right angle in front ; in the *second*, the right heel is placed against the middle of the left foot, forming a right angle both in front and in the rear ; in the *third*, the right heel is placed in front of the toes of the left foot in such a manner that the right foot points to the right ; in the *fourth*, the points of the feet are turned toward each other, and the heels are turned out as far as

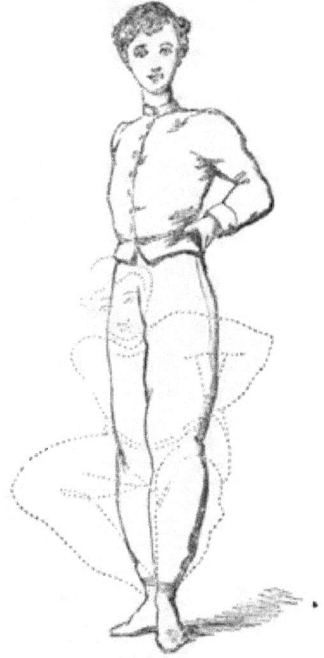

FIG. 75.

---

[1] **First Series.**—The movements of this Series are calculated to give strength and elasticity to the feet and legs, and, indirectly, ease, grace, and elegance to the whole carriage. They are also valuable preparatory exercises for walking, leaping, running, or dancing.

possible, so as to form nearly a straight line, as in Fig. 76. The *fifth*, *sixth*, and *seventh* positions correspond respectively to the *first*, *second*, and *third*, the heel of the left foot being behind that of the right in the *fifth* position, against the middle of the right foot in the *sixth*, and in front of the toes of the right foot in the *seventh*. In the *eighth* position[1] of Fig. 76, the heels are placed together, and the toes turned out, *so as to form a straight line*. In the *ninth*, the feet are placed about two inches apart, parallel, and pointed directly front, and the weight of the body is thrown upon the toes.

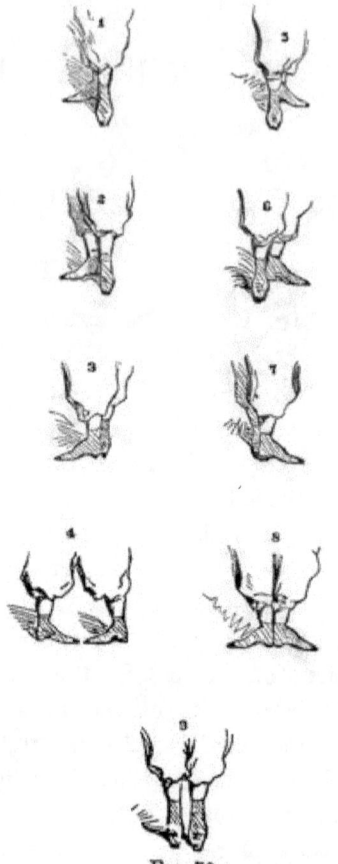

Fig. 76.

No. 155.—*First Movements*—Sink. At this command, the students sink as low as possible without throwing the feet out of position, as represented by the dotted part of Fig. 75, *the trunk remaining upright*, and then rise to their full height, four times, with the feet in each of the first four positions of Fig. 76. On each fourth upward motion, the next position of the feet is immediately taken *with a stamp*, without words of command.

No. 156.—*Second Movements*—Sink. These movements only differ from those of No. 155 in being executed in the *fifth*, *sixth*, *seventh*, and *eighth* positions of Fig. 76.

No. 157.—*Third Movements*[2]—Sink. These movements are

---

[1] **Eighth Position.**—On first attempting to take this position, the student may not be able to throw the toes quite out to a straight line; and in this case they should be turned only as far as possible *without rendering the body unsteady*. A little practice, however, will enable almost any one to assume the position with ease and comfort.

[2] **Third Movements.**—This class of movements is effective for render-

executed from the position of Fig. 77, in which the feet are in the *ninth* position of Fig. 76, by first letting down the body as low as possible, as in the dotted part of Fig. 77, and then raising it on the toes to its full height sixteen times. The trunk of the dotted part of the Fig., however, inclines too much forward, as *it should retain its upright position during the entire exercise.* At first, the maintenance of a vertical position of the trunk is attended with some difficulty, as there is involuntarily a greater or less disposition to bending forward, caused by the changing of the center of gravity ; but this is soon overcome.

Second Position.

No. 158.—At the command, *Second—Position*, the student will take the position of Fig. 59, which is the commencing position for the two classes of movements immediately following.

No. 159.—*First Movements*—RIGHT. At this command, the student will first stamp

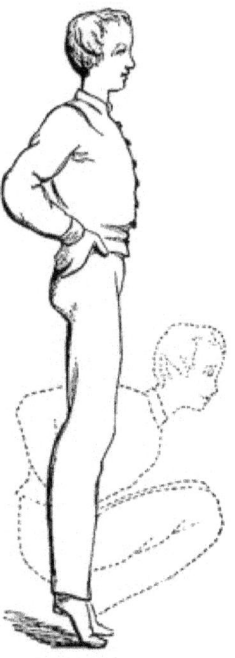

FIG. 77.

with the left foot, turning out its point as the commencing position is regained, and then immediately step to the right, with a stamp of the right foot, leaving about three times the length of the foot between the heels, thus taking the position of Fig. 78. In this position the toes are turned out so that the feet form nearly a straight line to the sides, and the body rests equally on both feet. As soon as this position is gained, the movements are continued by making the motion of the dotted part of Fig. 78, and regaining the position seven times. In making this motion to the right, the full weight of the body is thrown upon the right knee, *the left leg being kept rigid and straight.* As soon as the seventh change to the

---

ing freer all the joints of the leg and foot, though it chiefly employs the extensor muscles of the calves and toes. Owing to the exertion required to maintain the trunk in an upright position, it also acts in a not unimportant manner upon the lower muscles of the back.

right is made, the student instantly recovers the position of No. 158, by placing the right foot beside the left in the military position; then, at the command, LEFT, the student first stamps with the right foot and then steps to the left, with a stamp of the left foot, and makes seven motions to the left corresponding to the dotted part of Fig. 78, after which the original position is immediately regained.

No. 160.—*Second Movements*—ALTERNATE. At this command, the student, first stepping to the right with a stamp of the right foot, and then to the left with a stamp of the left foot, thus placing the heels about three times the length of the foot apart, makes seven of the motions of Fig. 78 by alternation, first to the right from this position and then to the left, when, at the command, BOTH, sixteen of these motions are described completely over from side to side, the body pausing in a vertical position only after the sixteenth outward motion has been made, when the position of No. 158 is instantly resumed.

No. 161.—*Third Movements*—RIGHT. This class of movements only differs from No. 159 in being exe-

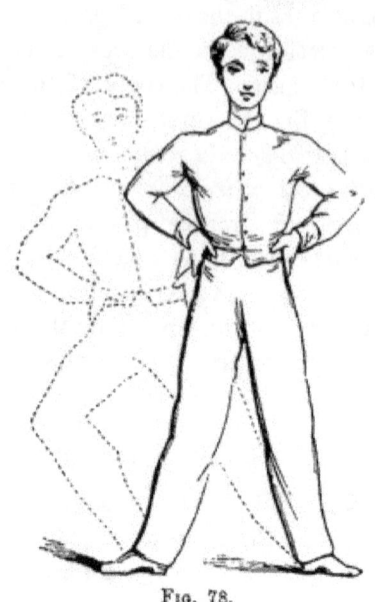

Fig. 78.

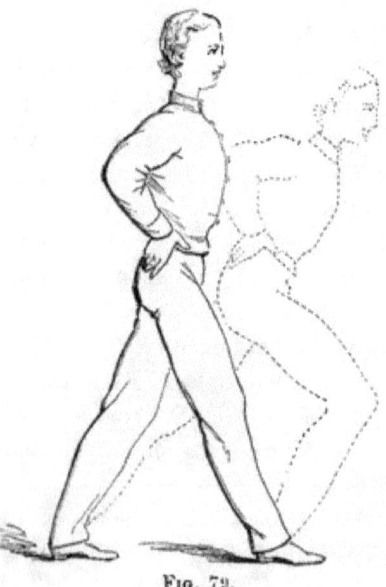

Fig. 79.

cuted directly front, as represented in Fig. 79. *The foot in the rear, however, should be turned sidewise instead of front.* In making the advanced movements of Fig. 79, the weight of the body is thrown wholly upon the forward foot, over which the knee is extended as far as possible, the trunk and the leg in the rear forming a straight line which inclines toward the horizontal floor.

SECOND SERIES.

First Position.

No. 162.—The instructor will command: 1. *Knee Exercise;* 2. *Second Series;* 3. *First*—POSITION.

No. 163.—At the last command, the student will take the position of Fig. 80, in which the knee is bent as much as possible, and pointed directly down, the calf of the leg and the heel being pressed firmly against the thigh.

No. 164.—*First Movements*— RIGHT. At this command, the right leg will first be straightened, and the right foot carried directly down and placed beside the left in the *military* position, p. 10, when the commencing position will immediately be regained. On the fourth motion from the commencing position, at the command, LEFT, the right foot will remain down, and the left leg will take a position corresponding to that of Fig. 80, when four downward motions will be made

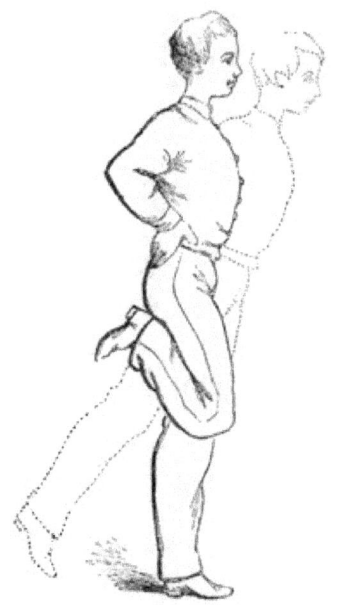

FIG. 80.

with the left leg and foot, on the last of which the right leg regains the position of Fig. 80; then, at the command, ALTERNATE, four downward motions will be made by alternation, the foot that sustains the body remaining in position until the descending one is placed by its side; and finally, at the command, RECIPROCATE, eight downward reciprocating motions will be made by springing from the floor, one foot taking the position at the same time the other one descends.

No. 165.—*Second Movements*—Right. At this command, the student will first make the motion of the dotted part of Fig. 80, by a vigorous kick with the right leg and foot, four times; then, at the command, Left, four corresponding backward motions will be made with the left leg and foot; and finally, at the command, Alternate, eight of these motions to the rear will be made with the right leg and the left alternately.

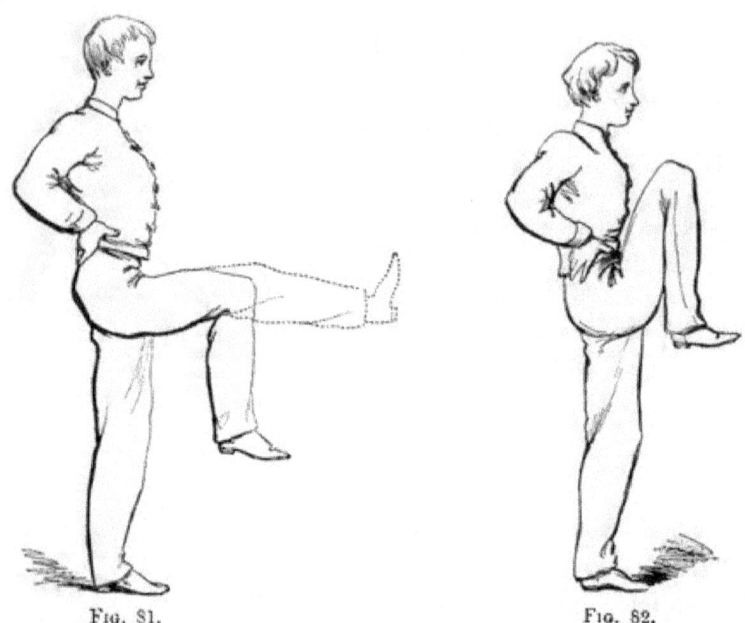

Fig. 81. Fig. 82.

No. 166.—*Third Movements (Combined)*—Right. The third class of movements is formed by a combination of the first and second classes. The right leg and foot first describe four of the motions of No. 164, from the position of Fig. 80; then four of the motions of No. 165; and finally, eight motions are made from the position alternately, the first being down and back to the original position, and the second to the rear. At the command, Left, the left leg and foot describe the same number of corresponding motions in combination.

Second Position.

No. 167.—At the command, *Second*—Position, the student will take the position of Fig. 81, in which the knee is raised front as high

KNEE EXERCISE.

as the hip. The *first, second,* and *third* classes of movements from this position correspond respectively to those of the position immediately preceding, the motions of the *first* being made directly down; of the *second,* directly out, as represented by the dotted part of Fig. 81; and of the *third,* by a combination of the *first* and the *second.*

No. 168.—*Fourth Movements*—Right. At this command, *from the position of Fig.* 81, the student first raises the right knee as high as possible, as in Fig. 82, and resumes the commencing position four times; then the right foot is brought down by the side of the left, and the knee raised to the commencing position four times; then, at the command, Alternate, four of these motions are made from the commencing position alternately, first up, as in Fig. 82; and finally, at the command, Both, eight motions are made the whole distance from the breast to the floor, the first commencing from, and the eighth terminating at, the position of Fig. 81.[1] At the command, Left, the left leg and foot describe the same number of corresponding motions.

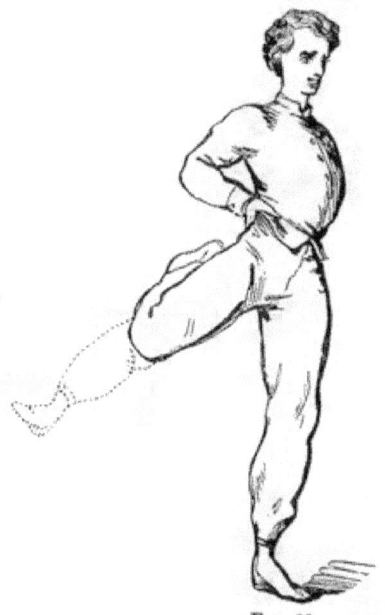

Fig. 83.

Third Position.

No. 169.—At the command, *Third*—Position, the student will take the position of Fig. 83. The *first, second,* and *third* classes of movements from this position correspond respectively to those of the Second Position, p. 100, the motions of the *first* being made directly down; of the *second,* directly sidewise, as represented by the dotted leg of Fig. 83; and of the *third,* by a combination of the *first* and the *second.* These movements will be made vigorously, but in slow time.

---

[1] These Movements become so perfect, after a fair amount of practice, that the knee lightly touches the breast on every upward motion; *the upper part of the body being kept as immovable as possible.*

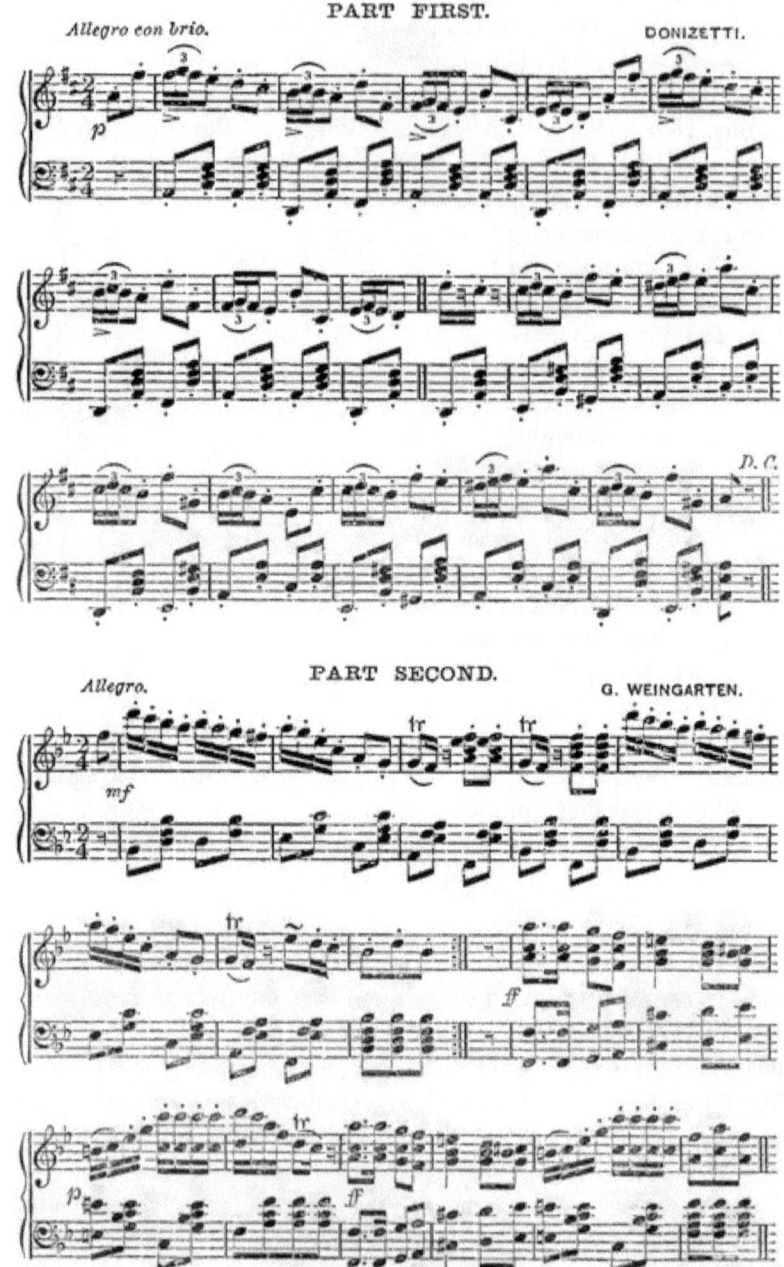

PART THIRD.

H. B. DODWORTH.

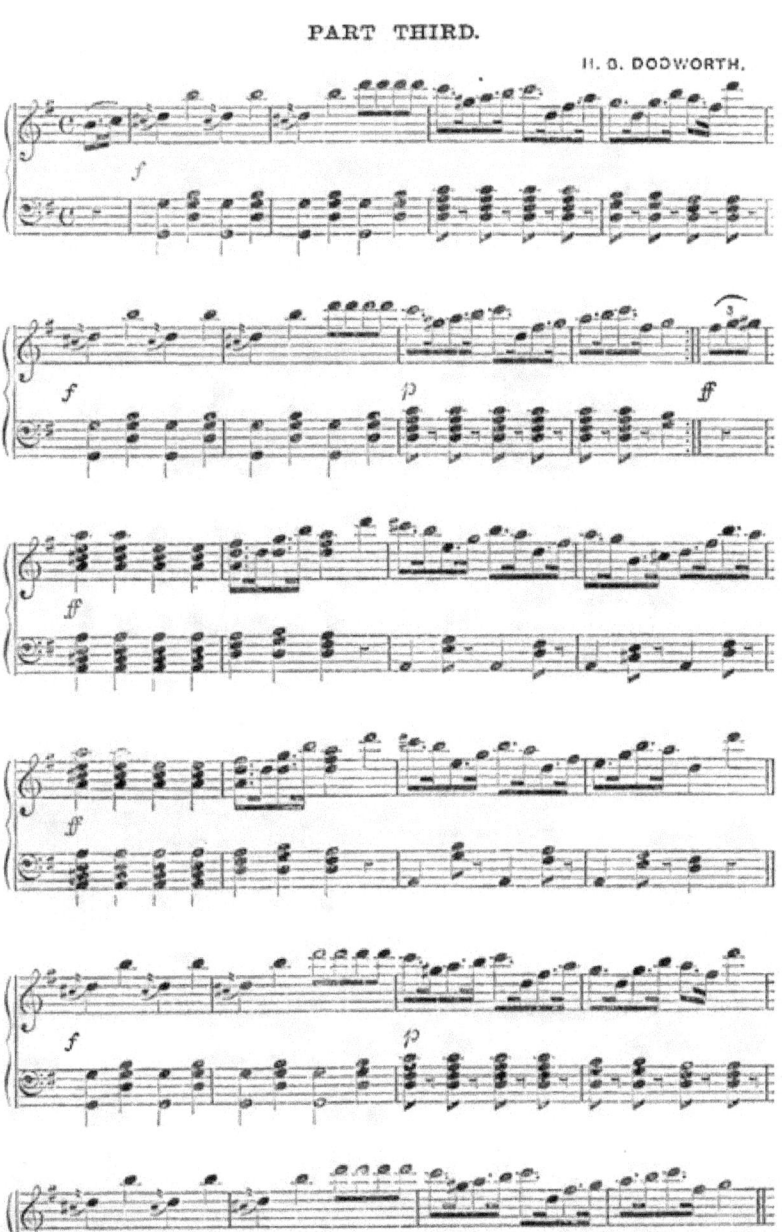

PART FOURTH.

C. A. MORRA.

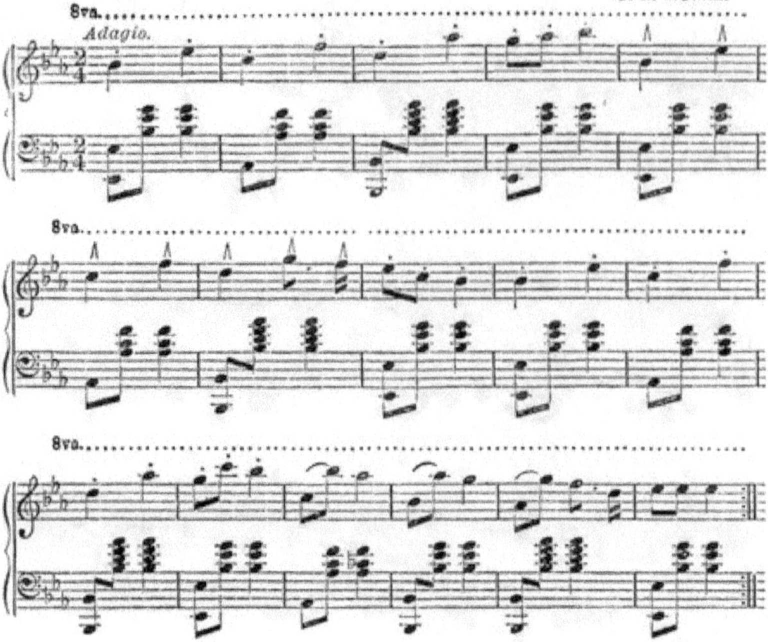

PART FIFTH.

VON WEBER.

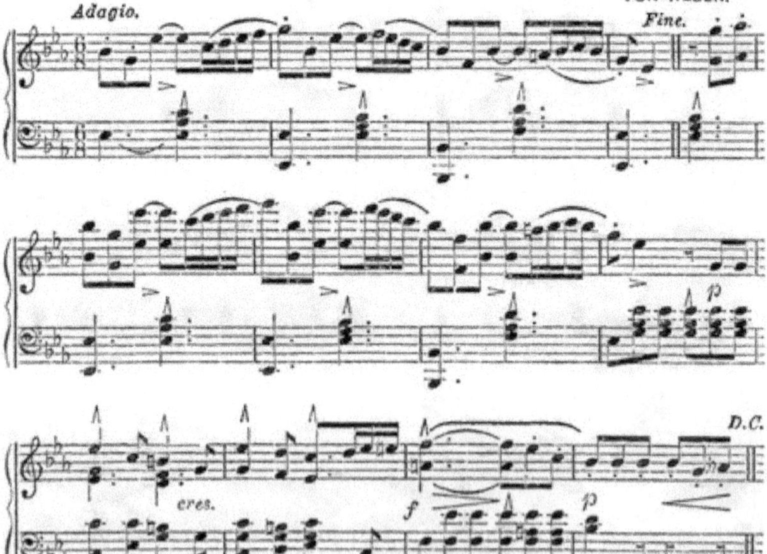

LEG AND FOOT EXERCISE.

PART SIXTH.

KUHNER.

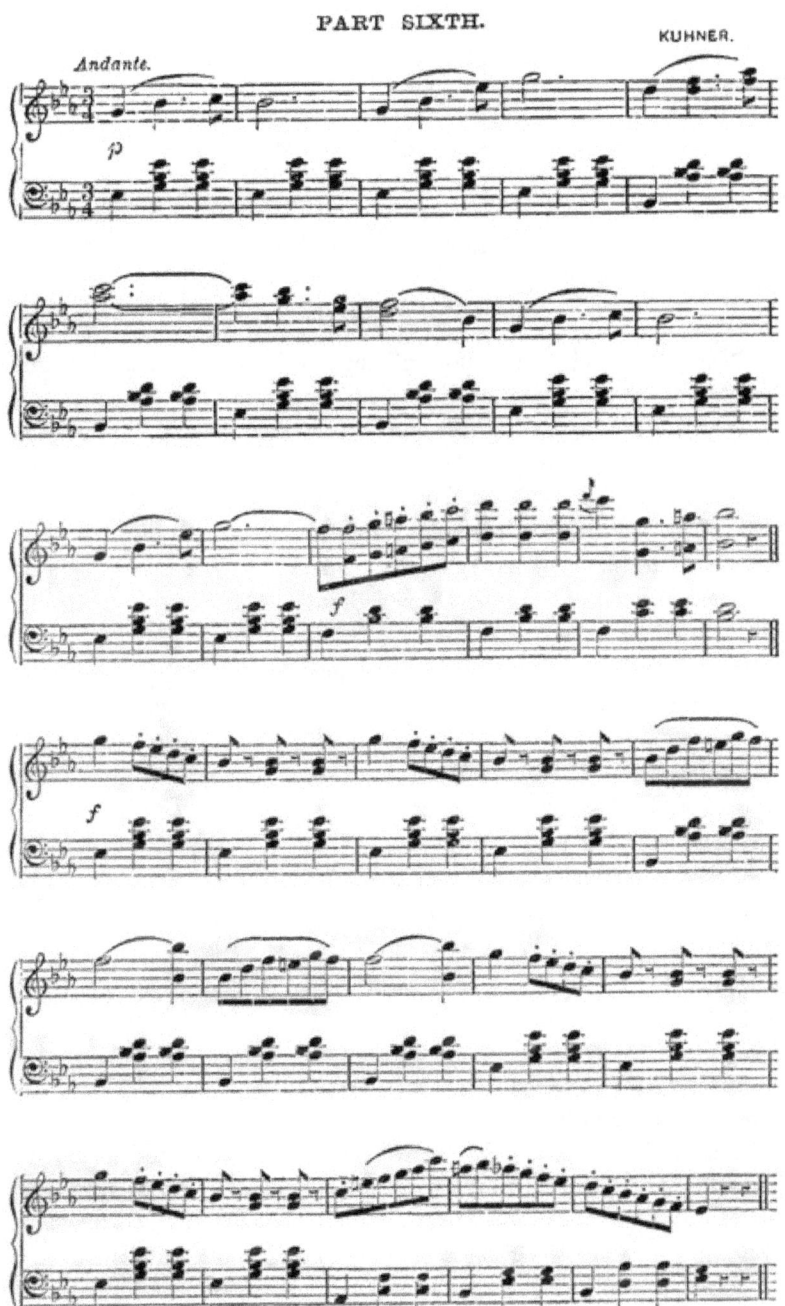

VIII.

LEG AND FOOT EXERCISE.

FIRST SERIES.

First Position.

No. 170.—The instructor will command: 1. *Leg and Foot Exercise;* 2. *First Series;* 3. *First*—Position.

No. 171.—At the third command, the student will take the position of Fig. 84.

No. 172.—*First Movements*—Right. First, the front part of the right foot will be raised and lowered eight times, as energetically as possible, as in Fig. 84, both an upward and a downward motion being made on each number counted; then, at the command, Left, the same number of corresponding motions will be made with the front part of the left foot; then, at the command, Alternate, eight of these motions will be made alternately, first with the right foot and then with the left; and finally, at the command, Reciprocate, eight of these motions will be made by reciprocation, the front of the right foot descending at the same time the front of the left foot ascends. During these movements the heels remain fixed, and the knees are held rather stiff.

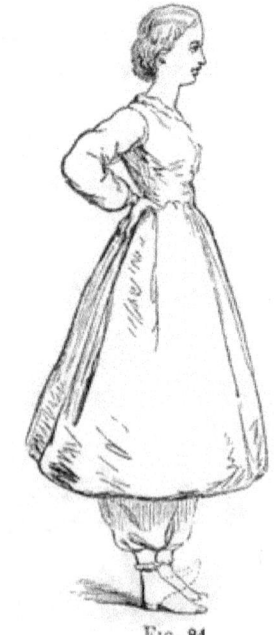

Fig. 84.

No. 173.—*Second Movements*—Right. These movements are described with the heels, the toes remaining fixed, while the remainder of the foot is raised and lowered as energetically as possible, as in Fig. 85. The knees will move freely. The remaining commands, and the number and order of the movements, are the same as in No. 172.

No. 174.—*Third Movements*—Toes. At this command, the fronts of both feet will be elevated and lowered four times simultaneously, as in Fig. 84; then, at the command, Heels, both heels will be raised and lowered four times simultaneously, as in Fig. 85; and finally, at the command, Alternate, eight of these double motions will be made alternately, the fronts of both feet being first raised and lowered, and then the heels. This class of movements is executed in slow time, both the upward and the downward motions being made on even numbers, or accented syllables.

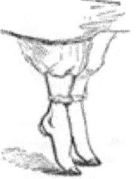

Fig. 85.

Second Position.

No 175.—*Second*—Position. At this command, the student will take the position of Fig. 86.

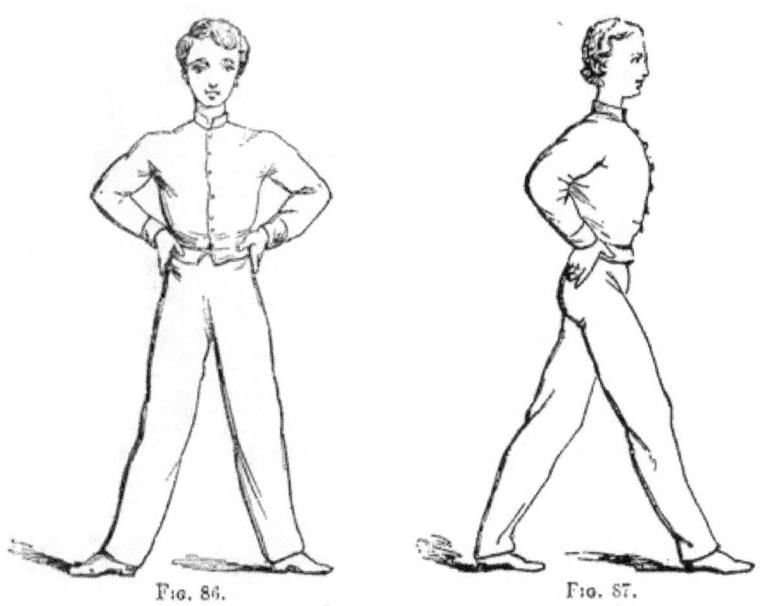

Fig. 86.   Fig. 87.

No. 176.—*First Movements*—Right. The remaining commands, and the number and order of the motions, are the same as in No. 172, the movements being made in the position of Fig 86. The *Second Movements* of this position correspond to No. 173; and the *Third*, to No. 174.

Third Position.

No. 177.—*Third*—Position. At this command, the student will take the position of Fig. 87. The commands, and the number and order of motions of the three classes of movements of this position, correspond respectively to those of the First Position, p. 106. After the movements have been executed with the right foot forward, as in Fig. 87, at the command, Change, the Third Position will be taken with the left foot forward, and the three classes of movements will be repeated.

SECOND SERIES.

First Position.

No. 178.—The instructor will command: 1. *Leg and Foot Exercise;* 2. *Second Series;* 3. *First*—Position.

No. 179.—At the last command, the student will take the position, by slightly elevating the toes and turning quickly on the heels, so that the inner parts of the feet touch each other from the heels to the toes, as in Fig. 88.

No. 180.—*First Movements*—Right At this command, the right foot will turn on the heel to the right, the point of the foot describing the arc A B in Fig. 88, so as to form a right-angle front with the heels, and recover the commencing position four times; then, at the command, Left, the left foot will make four corresponding outward motions from the position, describing the arc A C; and finally, at the command, Alternate, eight outward motions will be made with the feet alternately, the right foot first describing the arc A B and recovering the commencing position, and then the left foot describing the arc A C in like manner.

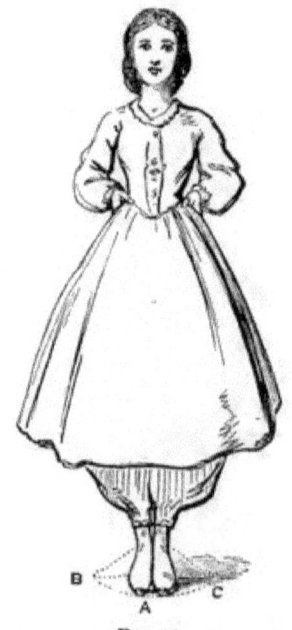

Fig. 88.

No. 181.—*Second Movements*—Right. The remaining commands, the number of motions, and the order in which they are made, are the same as in No. 180 ; but the toes are kept in position, and the heels are turned out sidewise as far as possible.

No. 182.—*Third Movements*—Toes. At this command, the points of both feet will be turned out simultaneously to the sides, describing the arcs A B and A C, Fig. 88, and brought back to the commencing position four times ; then, at the command, Heels, four outward motions will be made with the heels simultaneously ; and finally, at the command, Alternate, eight outward and inward motions will be made alternately, the points of both feet being first turned out to the sides and brought back to the commencing position, and then the heels. The time is marked by the patter of the toes, or the heels, on every outward or inward motion.

Second Position.

No. 183.—At the command, *Second*—Position, the position will be taken by first rising on the toes and springing into the air, and then instantly spreading the feet, dropping down upon the toes, and planting the feet twice the length of the student's foot apart, as in Fig. 89. *On every motion from, as well as to, this position, the foot is brought to the floor.*

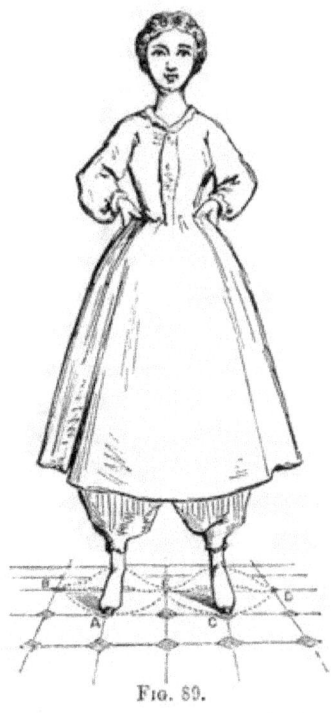

Fig. 89.

No. 184.—*First Movements*—Right. At this command, the front of the right foot is raised, and the foot is turned on the heel to the right, describing the arc A B, Fig. 89, and returned to the commencing position four times. The front of the foot beats the floor every time it arrives at the points B and A. At the command, Left, the left foot will describe the arc C D, in like manner, and recover the commencing position four times ; then, at the command, Alternate, four of these outward motions will be made with the feet alternately, the right foot first describing the arc A B and recovering the commencing position, and then the left foot, the arc C D; and finally, at the command, BOTH, the arcs A B and C D will be described with both feet simultaneously, and the commencing position regained, four times.

No. 185.—*Second Movements.*—RIGHT. The remaining commands, and the number and order of the motions, are the same as in No. 184; but this class of movements is executed by turning the feet *in*, thus describing the arcs A E and C E, Fig. 89.

No. 186.—*Third Movements*—OUT. At this command, both feet simultaneously turn on the heels to the right and left, describing the arcs A B and C D, Fig. 89, and regain the commencing position four times; then, at the command, IN, four corresponding simultaneous motions are made by turning the feet *in*, thus describing the arcs A E and C E; then, at the command, ALTERNATE, four combined motions from the position are made alternately, the toes first describing simultaneously the arcs A B and C D, and recovering the commencing position, and then the arcs A E and C E; and finally, at the command, BOTH, eight double motions will be made, the toes first describing the arcs A B and C D simultaneously, and then the entire arcs B A E and D C E, only stopping at the points A and C on the eighth motion.

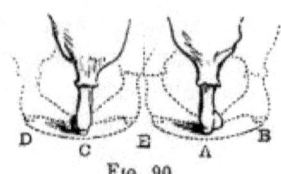

Fig. 90.

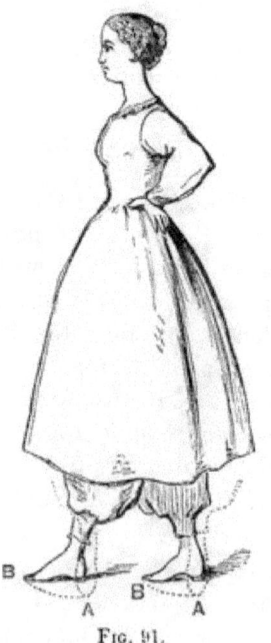

Fig. 91.

No. 187.—*Fourth, Fifth,* and *Sixth Movements.* These three classes of movements, which are described with the heels, as represented in Fig. 90, correspond respectively to those of Nos 184, 185, and 186, the *fourth,* being executed in the arcs A B and C D, Fig. 90; the *fifth,* in the arcs A E and C E; and the *sixth,* in the combined arcs A B and C D, A E and C E. During the execution of these movements, the toes will remain fixed at the points A and C, Fig. 89.

No. 188.—*Seventh Movements*—RIGHT. The seventh class of movements from the position of Fig. 89, is executed by turning the whole body on both heels to the right, describing simultaneously the arcs A B, A B, Fig. 91, and recovering the commencing position four times; then, at the command, LEFT, four corresponding motions from the position will be made to the left; then, at the command, ALTERNATE, four motions will be made from the position alternately, first to the right and back to the original position, and then to the left; and finally, at the command, BOTH, eight motions will be described the entire distance from right to left, the first motion commencing from, and only the eighth terminating at, the commencing position.

No. 189.—*Eighth Movements*—RIGHT. The remaining commands, and the number and order of the motions, are the same as in No. 188; *but the body turns on the toes*, the heels describing the arcs A B and G D, A D and C E, Fig. 92.

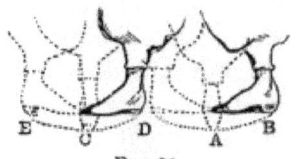

FIG. 92.

Third Position.

No. 190.—*Third*—POSITION. At this command, the student will take the military position, p. 10, which only differs from that of Fig. 93 in having the left heel brought down beside the right.

No. 191.—*First Movements (Facings)*—RIGHT. Facings are those movements by which the body turns upon its longitudinal axis so as to change its front direction. Each calisthenic facing consists in the body being turned to the *right* (describing one-fourth of a circle, as represented by the dotted part of Fig. 93) on the *left* heel, or to the *left* on the *right* heel, with the body kept perfectly upright. *The same heel that is used as a pivot to describe a side facing, is the one upon which the body is turned to the front, or to the commencing position.* Both feet will *tell the*

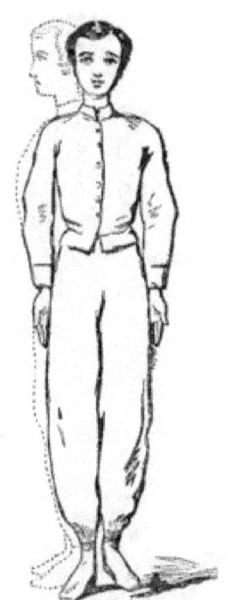

FIG. 93.

time as they come into a new position, or resume the commencing one. At the command, RIGHT, the student will raise the right foot slightly—just enough to clear the floor—turn on the left heel (raising the toes a little) until he faces exactly to the right; then, at the same instant, he will bring the toes of the left foot down, and the right foot to its place beside the left; heels together and toes turned out, as at first. The student will immediately regain the commencing position at the command, FRONT, or without a word of command. The facing to the right will be executed four times; then, at the command, LEFT, four corresponding facings will be executed to the left; and finally, at the command, ALTERNATE, eight facings will be executed alternately, first to the right and back to the front, and then to the left.

No. 192.—*Second Movements (Circles).* At the command, RIGHT, the student will describe two complete circles, each one of which is done in four facings or motions, the first being to the right, the second to the rear, the third to the rear of the right, and the fourth regains the commencing position; then, at the command, LEFT, two inverse circles will be described to the left; and finally, at the command, ALTERNATE, four alternate circles will be described in like manner, the first to the right, the second to the left, &c. The motions commencing to the *right* will be made on the *left* heel, and those to the *left*, on the *right* heel.

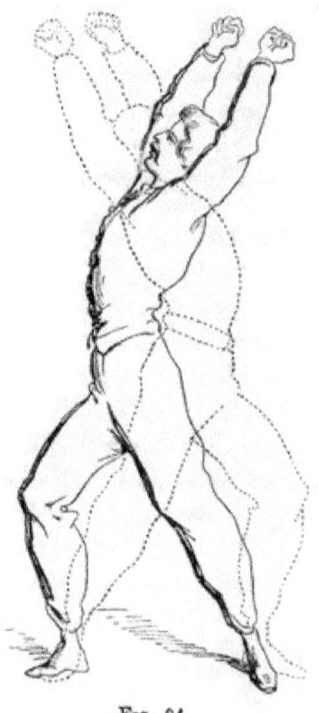

FIG. 94.

No. 193.—*Third Movements (About)*—FACE. Unlike military facings, the full face to the rear will be executed on but one heel at a time. The remaining commands, and the number and order of these circles, are the same as in No. 192; *but every facing or motion describes one-half of a circle.* The motions of this class are only made on even numbers or accented syllables. At the termination of each motion, the fronts of the feet come down with a slight *stamp*, to mark the time. In executing the facings, *the student will keep the body erect, the arms from swinging, and the head firm in its place, without looking down.*

Fourth Position.

No. 194.—*Fourth*—POSITION. At this command, the student will take the fourth position, which only differs from the military position, p. 10, in placing the heels two and one-half times the length of the student's foot apart, and shutting the hands.

No. 195.—*First Movements*—RIGHT. The first and only class of movements from this position is formed by the combined action of nearly all the muscles of the body. At the command, RIGHT, a facing is executed by simultaneously turning on both heels to the right, straightening the left leg, throwing the whole weight of the body on the right knee, energetically raising both arms and projecting the chest, as represented in Fig. 94. First, this outward motion is made to the right, and the commencing position resumed four times; then, at the command, LEFT, four corresponding motions from the position are made to the left; then, at the command, ALTERNATE, four of these outward motions from the position are made to the right and left alternately; and finally, at the command, BOTH, eight motions are made in combination from side to side, as represented in Fig. 94, the first commencing *from*, and only the eighth terminating *at*, the commencing position.

THIRD SERIES.

First Position.

No. 196.—The instructor commands: 1. *Leg and Foot Exercise;* 2. *Third Series;* 3. *First*—POSITION.

No. 197.—On the word, POSITION, the student will take the position of Fig. 95, in which the weight of the body is sustained by the point of the left foot, and the right leg and point of the foot are held out to the right, both knees being kept rather stiff. This position, however, is taken in four directions during the execution of the movements.

No. 198.——*First Movements*[1]—
RIGHT. At this command, the student will raise and sink the front of the extended foot as far as possible, as in Fig. 95, eight times. On the eighth upward motion, the command, LEFT, will be given, and the student will instantly take his position to the left, by sustaining the weight of the body upon the point of the right foot, and extending the left leg and foot to the left, when eight upward and downward motions will be made with the front of the left foot. If the student find it too difficult, he will not at first be restricted to the *point* of the sustaining foot. In connection with the movements of this position, which take place simply by means of the ankle joint, there should be also an energetic bending and stretching of the toes. Thus the muscles of the shin and calf, as well as the lower part of the thigh, and the foot, are brought into play.

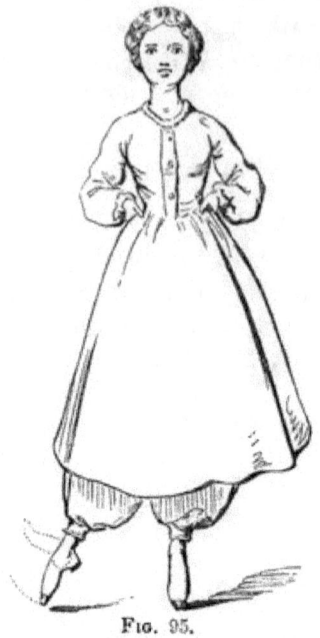

FIG. 95.

No. 199.—*Second Movements (Front)*—RIGHT. The remaining commands, and the number, order, and kind of motions, are the same as in No. 198; but first the right leg, and then the left, are extended front, inclining toward the floor at an angle of nearly 45 degrees, instead of to the sides.

---

[1] **Movements.**—At first, the student will find it difficult to keep his balance while executing the movements of this Series, especially those of No. 200; but he must learn to do so without leaning upon any thing, because otherwise a great part of the effect of the compound working is lost. This very endeavor to keep one's balance and the upright position of the body, calls into action many muscles, and is one of the aims of the exercise. The movements sidewise, and forward and backward, require the working of the muscular parts all round, and from all sides of the hips. They also have an effect upon all the muscles of the legs and feet; for the leg, apparently so immovable, has enough to do to maintain the equilibrium of the body, menaced from so many sides.

Second Position.

No. 200.—*Second*—POSITION. This position only differs from the military position, p. 10, in having the right foot raised about two inches from the floor, and the hands fixed upon the hips, with the thumbs front.

No. 201.—*First Movements*—RIGHT. At this command, the right leg is extended sidewise to the point A, Fig. 96, from whence it describes the arc A B four times; then, at the command, CHANGE, the right foot is brought back into position, and the left leg is extended left to the point B, from which it describes the arc B A four times; then, at the command, CHANGE, the position of Fig. 96 is resumed, and the right leg describes the arc A B *behind* the left leg four times; and finally, the command CHANGE is again given, and the left leg describes the arc B A *behind* the right leg four times from the point B.

No. 202.—*Second Movements*—RIGHT. At this command, the right leg is extended sidewise to the point A, Fig. 96, from whence it describes the arc A B four times, in front of the left leg; four times, behind the left leg; and finally, eight times alternately, first in front of the left leg, and then behind it. At

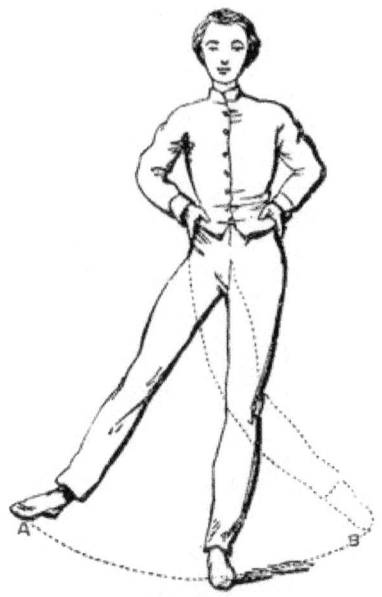

FIG. 96.

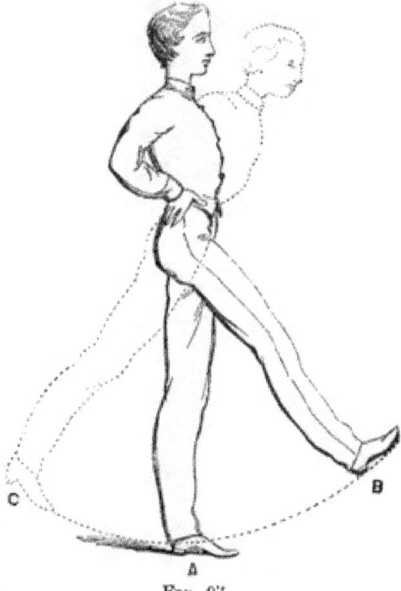

FIG. 97.

the command, LEFT, the left leg is extended to the point B, from whence it describes the same number of corresponding motions.

No. 203.—*Third Movements*—RIGHT. With both feet in position at A, Fig. 97, at this command the right foot will be thrown directly forward to the point B, and back to the commencing position, four times; then the same foot will describe the arc A C, and recover the commencing position four times; and finally, this foot will be thrown forward to the point B, from whence it will describe the entire arc B A C, without bending either leg, eight times. At the command, LEFT, the right foot will sustain the weight of the body, and the left leg and foot will describe the same number of corresponding motions, in like order.

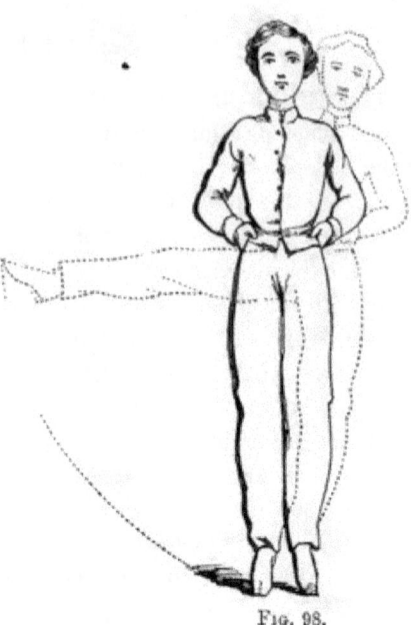

FIG. 98.

Third Position.

No. 204.—At the command, *Third*—POSITION, the students take the position of Fig. 98, in which the weight of the body is sustained by the toes.

No. 205.—*First Movements*—RIGHT. During the

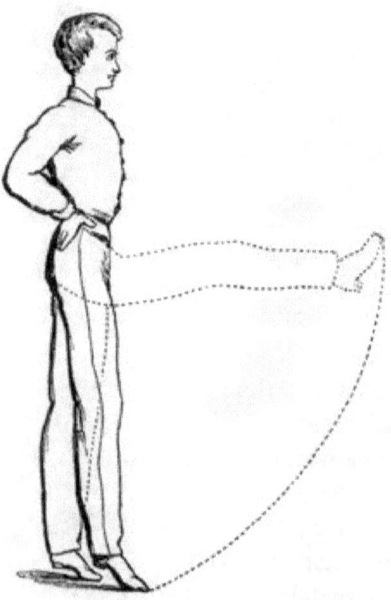

FIG. 99.

execution of these movements, both legs will be kept straight. At the first command, the student will raise the right leg sidewise so as to form a right angle, as in Fig. 98, and regain the commencing position four times; then, at the command, LEFT, the left leg will describe four corresponding motions from the position to the left; and finally, at the command, ALTERNATE, eight of these outward motions will be made to the right and left alternately.

No. 206.—*Second Movements*—RIGHT. The number and order of these movements are the same as in No. 205; but the motions are made directly front, as represented in Fig. 99.

FOURTH SERIES.

First Position.

No. 207.—The instructor commands: 1. *Leg and Foot Exercise;* 2. *Fourth Series;* 3. *First*—POSITION.

No. 208.—At the third command, the student will take the First Position, in which the weight of the body is supported chiefly by the point of the left foot, the point of the right foot being placed upon the floor at a moderate distance to the right of the left foot, as in Fig. 100.

No. 209.—*First Movements*—RIGHT. At this command, the right leg first will swing round in front of the left leg, the toes of the right foot being placed upon the floor at the point B, as represented by the dotted part of Fig. 100, and recover the commencing position at A four times; then the same number of corresponding motions will be made by the right leg *behind* the left, the point of the right foot touching the floor only at B and A; and finally, eight of these motions will be made from the point A alternately, the first in front of the

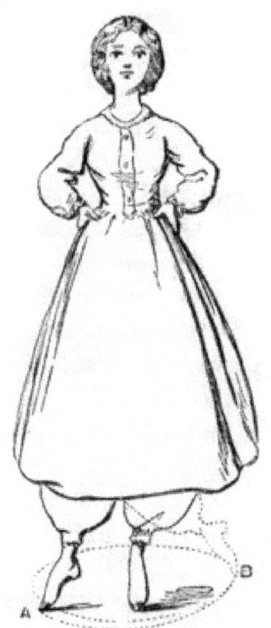

FIG. 100.

left leg, the second behind it, &c. At the command, LEFT, the position will be taken to the left, the weight of the body resting chiefly on the point of the right foot, and the left leg will describe the same number of corresponding motions around the right leg, and in like order.

No. 210.—*Second Movements*—RIGHT. At this command, from the position of Fig. 100, the right leg will swing round front, and the toes of the right foot will touch the floor at the point B, from whence complete circles around the left leg will be described back and front, the toes of the right foot touching every time they arrive at the point B. On the eighth motion, at the command, CHANGE, the position will be taken to the left, when the left leg will describe eight corresponding motions; and finally, eight of these motions will be made with each leg, *only touching the floor with the foot that is in motion at the command,* CHANGE.

Second Position.

No. 211.—At the command, *Second*—POSITION (*Foot Circles*), the student will take the position of Fig. 101, in which the right leg is first extended to the right, and the weight of the body supported on the left foot.

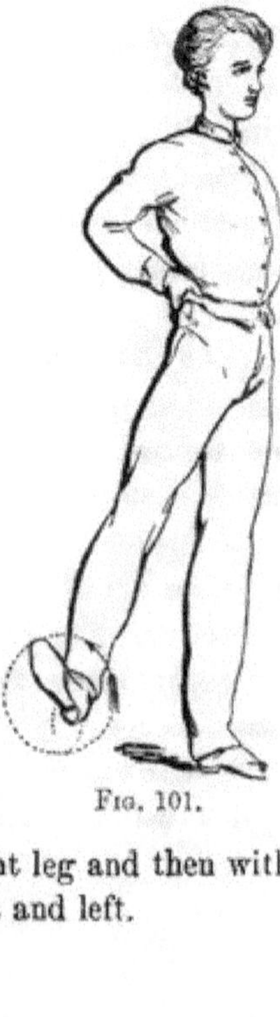

No. 212.—*First Movements*—RIGHT. At this command, eight circles will be described with the point of the right foot, in the direction indicated by the arrow in Fig. 101, and then the same number of like circles in a contrary direction; then, at the command, CHANGE, the position will be taken to the left, and the left foot will describe the same number of corresponding back and front circles. In executing the movements of this position, the extended leg describes small circles, though the foot circles are chiefly formed by the motion of the ankle-joint, and an energetic bending and stretching of the toes.

No. 213.—*Second Movements*. The remaining commands, and the number and order of the movements, are the same as in No. 212; but the position is taken in front, first with the right leg and then with the left, and the circles are described to the right and left.

FIG. 101.

Third Position.

No. 214.—At the command, *Third—Position*, the student will take the position by extending the right leg, first to the right, as in Fig. 102.

No. 215.—*First Movements*—Right. The remaining commands, and the number, order, and directions of the two classes of movements of this position, are the same as those of the Second Position of this Series. In executing these movements, both to the sides and in front, *the extended leg will be kept perfectly straight*, and the circles will be made as high and large as possible, as represented in Figs. 102 and 103. The trunk, also, will be kept as immovable as possible. The student will practice these movements frequently, and become as perfect in their execution as possible, as they render freër the play of the legs in their sockets, and set in active motion all the mus-

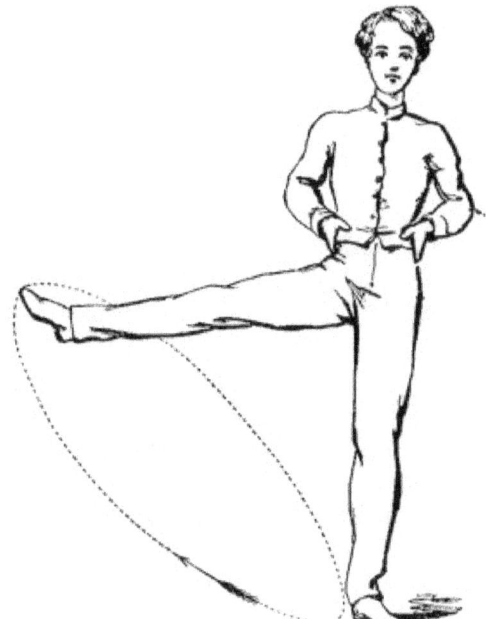

Fig. 102.

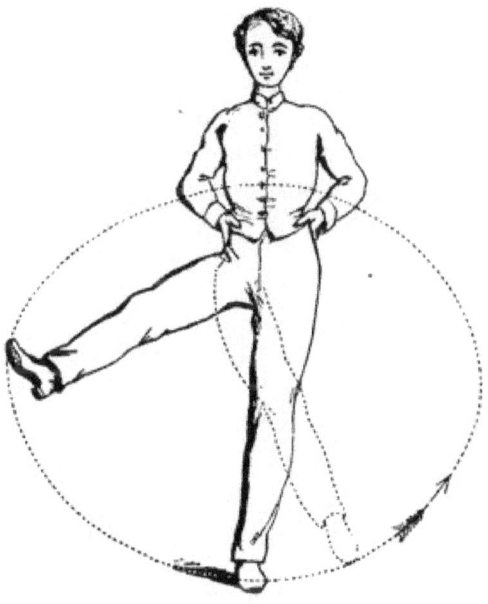

Fig. 103.

cles of the trunk, especially those of the back and loins, as well as the allotment muscles of the legs.

FIFTH SERIES.

First Position.

No. 216.—The instructor will command: 1. *Leg and Foot Exercise;* 2. *Fifth Series;* 3. *First*—POSITION.

No. 217.—At the third command, the student will take the position of Fig. 104, which only differs from the *military* position, p. 10, in supporting the weight of the body with the point of the right foot, the left foot being elevated about two inches from the floor.

No. 218.—*First Movements.* The first and only class of movements is executed by hopping in place, first four times on the point of the right foot; then four times on the point of the left foot; then eight times in alternate double hops, the first and second being on the right foot, the second and third on the left, &c.; and finally, sixteen times by a reciprocating motion, the point of one foot passing to the floor at the same time the other springs from it. The instructor will at first employ the commands of execution, RIGHT, LEFT, ALTERNATE, RECIPROCATE, while the students count, using the first variety on p. 40. These leaps are made by springing directly up into the air without spreading the feet, or swaying the arms or the upper part of the body. The trunk is kept vertical throughout the exercise.

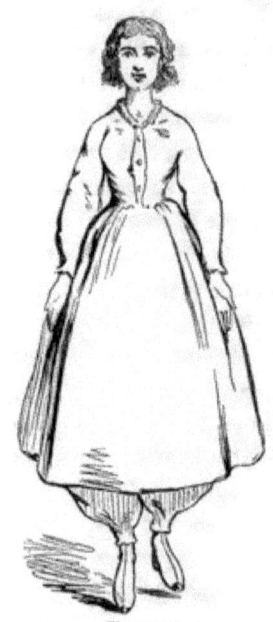

FIG. 104.

Second Position.

No. 219.—*Second*—POSITION. At this command, the position will first be taken as represented in Fig. 105, by extending the right leg to the right, and supporting the weight of the body upon the very point of the left foot, *both legs being kept straight and rigid during the entire exercise, and the front of the extended foot being bent down as much as possible.*

No. 220.—*First Movements.* First spring into the air, and alight on the toes of the left foot sixteen times; then, at the command, CHANGE, take the position to the left, and hop from the point of the right foot sixteen times.—*Second Movements.* The position with each leg is taken to the front for this class, as in Fig. 106, the student first hopping sixteen times on the point of the left foot, and then on the right.— In executing the *Third Movements,* the position for each leg is taken to the rear, as represented by the dotted part of Fig. 106. Sixteen hops are taken on the point of each foot. Students will first practice these exercises in connection with counting, being careful not to leap too high, as a hop must be done on every number.

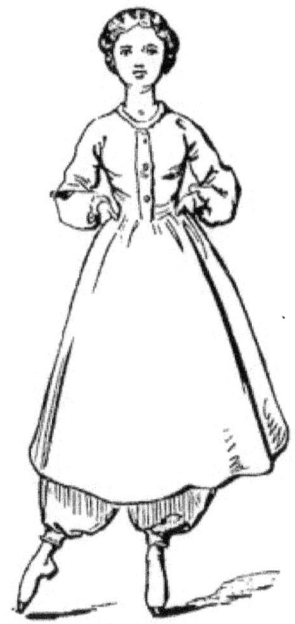

Fig. 105.

Third Position.

No. 221.—At the command, *Third*—POSITION, the student will take the position of Fig. 107, in which the entire weight of the body is supported by the points of the feet.

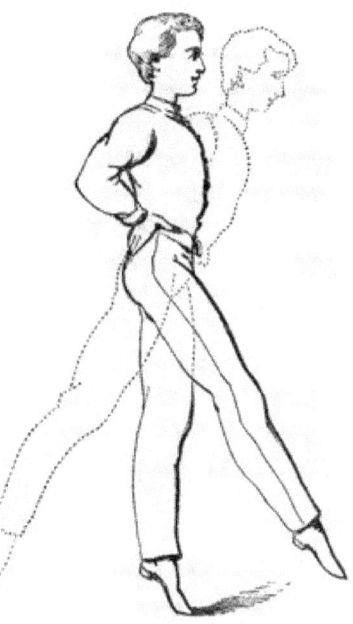

Fig. 106.

No. 222.—*First, Second, and Third Movements (Facings).* The commands, and number and order of motions that constitute these three classes of movements, correspond respectively to those of Nos. 191, 192, and 193; but the facings differ in being described on the toes by leaping, as in Fig. 107. *Every leap is executed in one time and two motions.* The student bends the knees, the weight of the body resting on the points of the feet, and instantly, by a sudden straightening of the knees and a vigorous action of the toes, springs into the air, and, having described the prescribed portion of a circle, alights upon the toes, as shown by the dotted part of Fig. 107. In executing the *Third Movements*, slow time will be employed, as one half of a circle is described at each leap.

No. 223.—*Fourth Movements*—Right. At this command, from the position of Fig. 107, the student will spring into the air, crossing the right leg in front of the left, alighting upon the points of the feet, as in Fig. 108, and immediately regain the commencing position four times; then, at the command, Left, the legs will be crossed in like manner, the *left* in front of the *right*, and the commencing position regained four times; then, at the command, Alternate, the legs will be crossed and the commencing position regained four times alternately; and finally, at the command, Reciprocate, eight leaps will be made, accompanied with a reciprocal crossing of the legs, the legs crossing each other on every leap, the right leg in front, as in Fig. 108, on the first leap, the left on the second, &c., only resuming the commencing position on the eighth leap.

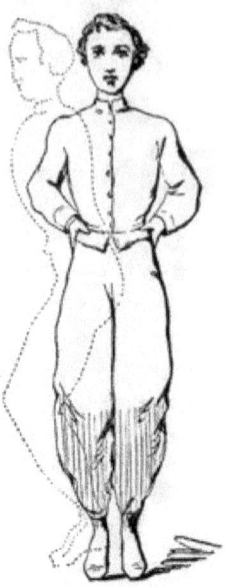

Fig. 107.

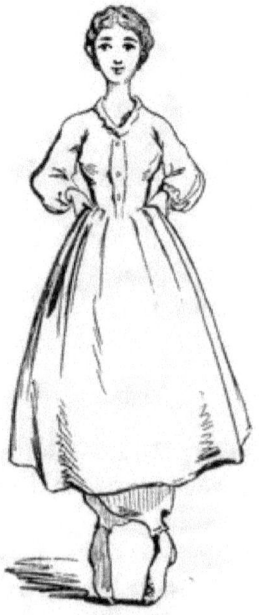

Fig. 108.

LEG AND FOOT EXERCISE. 123

SIXTH SERIES.

First Position.

No. 224.—The instructor will command: 1. *Leg and Foot Exercise;* 2. *Sixth Series;* 3. *First*—POSITION.

No. 225.—At the third command, the student will take the position of Fig. 109, in which the whole weight of the body is supported by the toes.

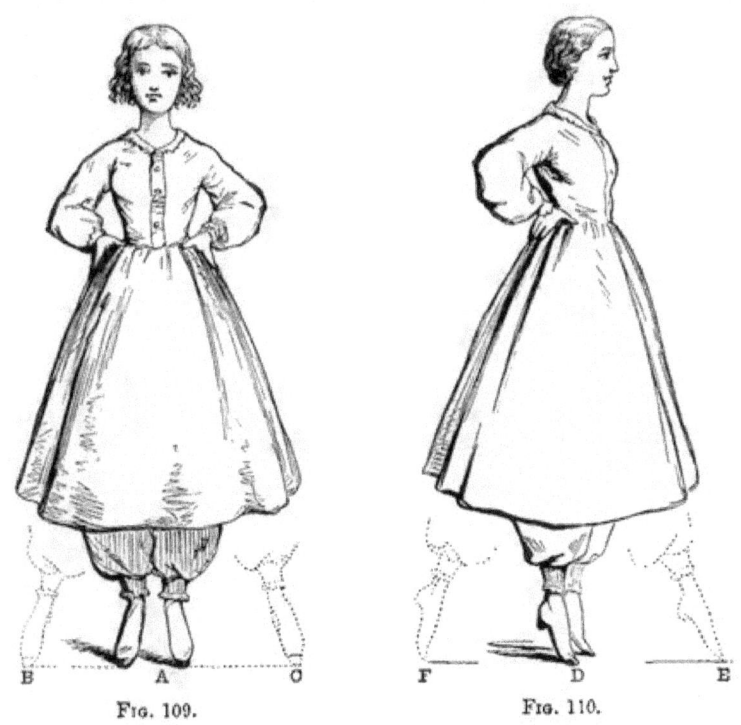

FIG. 109.   FIG. 110.

No. 226.—*First Movements (Sliding Toes).* All the movements of this position are executed without lifting the points of the feet from the floor or touching the heels. First, at the command, RIGHT, the point of the right foot describes the line A B, Fig. 109, and recovers the commencing position four times; then, at the command, LEFT, the point of the left foot describes the line A C, and recovers the commencing position four times; then, at the command, ALTERNATE, four of these motions from the position are made with the feet by alternation; and finally, at the command, BOTH, the lines A B and A C are described simultaneously, and the commencing position regained four times.

No. 227.—*Second and Third Movements.* The commands of execution are, RIGHT, LEFT, ALTERNATE, RECIPROCATE. The *Second Movements* are made by sliding the toes directly front in the line D E, Fig. 110. The right foot first passes to E, and regains the commencing position four times; then the left foot; then four of these motions from the position are made alternately; and finally, seven front motions are made by reciprocation (four with the right foot and three with the left), the left foot being advanced at the same time the right foot is regaining the commencing position, and conversely. *Third Movements.* These only differ from the second class of movements in being executed to the rear in the line D F, Fig. 110.

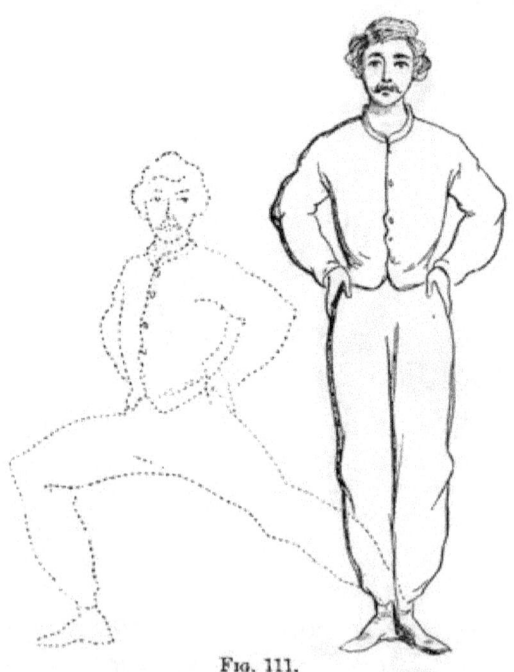

FIG. 111.

No. 228.—*Fourth, Fifth, and Sixth Movements.* These three classes of movements correspond respectively to the *First, Second,* and *Third,* the *Fourth* being executed in the lines A B and A C, Fig. 109; the *Fifth,* in the line D E, Fig. 110; and the *Sixth,* in the line

LEG AND FOOT EXERCISE.

D F. *The difference consists in executing the movements by lifting the feet and bearing them over the spaces, touching the toes only at the points* B, C, E, *and* F, *instead of sliding them.*

Second Position.

No. 229.—At the command, *Second*—POSITION, the student will take the position of Fig. 111.

No. 230.—*First Movements (Charges).* In executing charges, the student, with one foot fixed, takes strides as great as possible without preventing an easy recovery of the commencing position, in the direction prescribed. *The leg whose foot remains in position must be kept rigid and straight, and so turned upon the heel that the two feet are at right angles.* This class of movements is done by

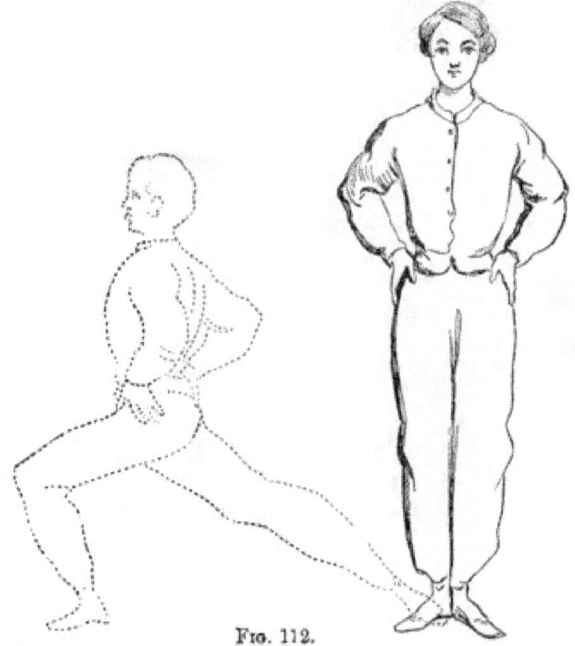

FIG. 112.

charging sidewise, first to the right with the right leg, as represented by the dotted part of Fig. 111, and regaining the commencing position four times; then a charge is done to the left with the left leg, and the commencing position regained four times; and finally, eight charges are made to the right and left alternately. The commands of execution are, RIGHT, LEFT, ALTERNATE.

No. 231.—*Second Movements.* These movements only differ from No. 230 in being made *directly front, left leg and foot first.*

No. 232.—*Third Movements.* The remaining commands, and the number and order of the motions, are the same as in No. 230; but the charges are made front, bearing toward the right and the left, at an angle of 45 degrees.

No. 233.—*Fourth Movements.* These movements are formed by combining facings and charges. The student, turning on the right heel, charges to the right with the left leg, thus executing a facing, as represented by the dotted part of Fig. 112, and recovers the commencing position four times; then four corresponding charges are made to the left with the right leg; and finally, eight of these charges are made to the right and left alternately.—The Music best adapted to the four classes of movements immediately preceding, will be found on pp. 85, 86, 104, and 105.

SEVENTH SERIES.

First Position.

No. 234.—The instructor will command : 1. *Leg and Foot Exercise;* 2. *Seventh Series;* 3. *First*—Position.

No. 235.—At the last command, the student takes the position of Fig. 114, which only differs from the *military* position, p. 10, in supporting the weight of the body upon the points of the feet.

No. 236.—*First Movements.* At the command, *First Movements*—Left; or, *Sidewise, Mark Time*—March, the student, facing the instructor, and standing in the position of Fig. 114, at the point A, Fig. 113, will step to the left, first planting the toes of the left foot at the point B, and lightly touching the side of the left foot with the right; then he will plant the toes of the right foot at the point c, slightly touching the right foot with the left, thus describing the motion shown in Fig. 113. This motion will be continued, without making progress forward, until thirty-two steps have been taken. At the command, Halt, or on the thirty-second step, the commencing position will be resumed at the point A. These steps will be taken at the rate of about ninety in a minute. While the students are counting to mark the time, as is prescribed on p. 40, in order to insure uniformity in the order of taking the step, the instructor will repeat the words, *Left—Right—Left—Right*, &c. When this swaying movement is described in columns, the students will *cover square*, that is, keep exactly behind those in the file front.

No. 237.—*Second Movements.* As soon as the student is sufficiently established in the principles of this step, at the command, *Second Movements*—Left; or, *Class, Forward*—March, he will advance with this swaying motion, first with the *left* foot at an angle of 45 degrees to the left, *planting flat the left foot*, and bringing the right foot to the left until it touches the left foot, then the right foot is thrown forward, bearing to the right at an angle of 45 degrees, and planted in like manner. When the instructor shall wish to arrest the march, he will command, *Class*—Halt. At the second word of this command, which will be given at the instant when either foot is coming to the ground, the foot in the rear will be brought up and planted by the side of the other.

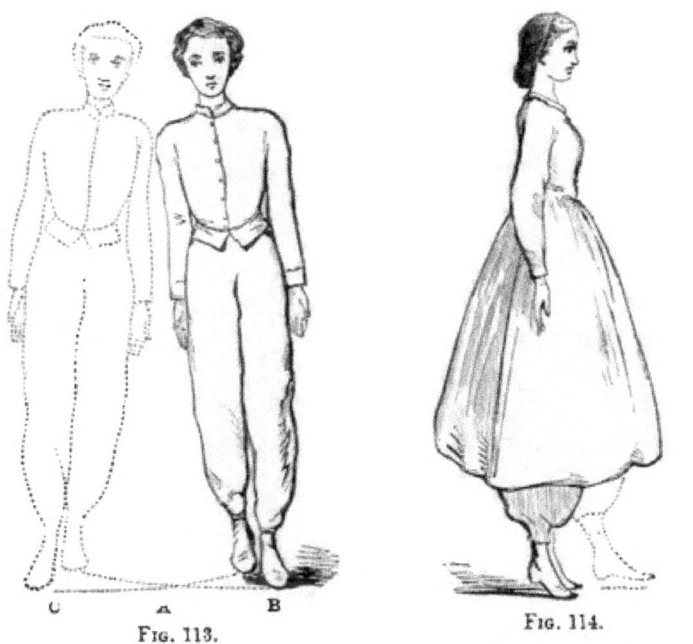

Fig. 113.   Fig. 114.

No. 238.—*Third Movements.* At the command, *Third Movements*—Left; or, *On Toes, Mark Time*—March, the left leg is first thrown forward as if to take a step, as shown by the dotted leg of Fig. 114, *without inclining the body forward in the least*, and brought back to its place, and then a corresponding motion is made with the right leg. These motions are continued without making progress until thirty-two steps are taken, or the command, *Class—* HALT, is given. The instructor will frequently require the student to execute these movements on the heels, without touching the fronts of the feet. The command is, *On Heels, Mark Time*—MARCH.— When the preparatory command, *On Toes*, or *On Heels*, is not given, the student will *mark time* from the *military* position, p. 10, planting the advanced foot flat every time it recovers the commencing position. As the feet are thrown front in executing these movements, they will be bent at the ankles so that the toes shall hang forward.

No. 239.—*Fourth Movements.* After the student has learned to *mark time perfectly*, remembering always *to start with the left foot first*, at the command, *Fourth Movements—*LEFT ; or, *Class, Forward; Common* (or *Quick*) *Time—*MARCH, he will smartly, but without a jerk, carry straight forward the left foot twenty-eight inches from the right (twenty inches for small boys and girls), the sole near the floor or ground, the ham extended, the point of the foot a little depressed, and, as also the knee, slightly turned out ; he will, at the same time, throw the weight of the body forward, and plant flat the left foot, without shock, precisely at the distance where it finds itself from the right when the weight of the body is brought forward, the whole weight of which will now rest upon the advanced foot. The student will next, in like manner, advance the right foot and plant it as above, the heel twenty-eight inches from the heel of the left foot, and thus continue to march without crossing the legs, or striking one leg against the other, without turning the shoulders, and preserving always the face direct to the front. At the command, *On Toes* (or *Heels*)—MARCH, without arresting the march, the students will march on their toes or heels without touching other portions of the feet. In *common time*, the student marches at the rate of ninety steps in a minute ; in *quick* time, at the rate of one hundred and ten steps per minute.—The best Music for marches will be found on pp. 48, 49, 54, 57, and 103.

Second Position.

No. 240.—*Second—*POSITION In this position, the arms are bent, with the elbows to the rear, the forearms against the waist, the hands closed, and the nails toward the body, as in Fig. 115; but the legs, when not in motion, are not bent at the knee as here represented. The trunk is inclined forward, the head slightly back.

No. 241.—*First Movements (Trotting Exercise)*—LEFT. At this command, the left leg will be thrown *back*, the weight of the body being supported on the point of the right foot, and brought to the commencing position, as represented by the dotted leg of Fig. 115; then a corresponding motion will be made with the right leg, and these alternate motions will be continued until thirty-two steps shall have been taken, at an average rate of one hundred and twenty to the minute. During these movements, the joints of the knee and ankle must be quite free and elastic, bending as in the common motion of trotting, though no progress is made. The degree of intensity of the movement can be regulated at will, by raising the foot to any desirable height.

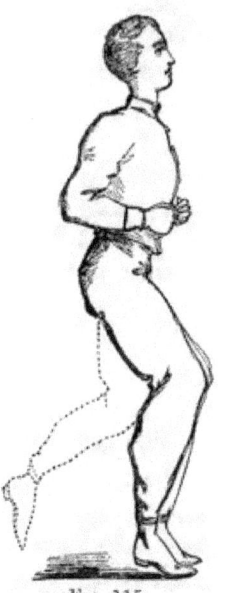

FIG. 115.

No. 242.—*Second Movements (Double Quickstep).* At the command, *Second Movements*—LEFT; or, *Mark Time, Double Quick*—MARCH, the student—with the feet in the *military* position, p. 10, and the arms in the position of Fig. 115,—will raise *to the front* his left leg bent, in order to give the knee the greatest elevation, the part of the leg between the knee and the instep vertical, the toe depressed; he will then replace his foot in its former position; with the right leg he will execute what has just been prescribed for the left, and the alternate movement of the legs will be continued until thirty-two steps are taken, or the instructor commands, *Class*—HALT. The rate of swiftness of this step is from one hundred and sixty-five to one hundred and eighty per minute.

No. 243.—*Third Movements.* These movements only differ from those of No. 242 in making progress from the spot. At the command, *Third Movements*—LEFT; or, *Class Forward, Double Quick*—MARCH, the student will carry forward the left foot, the leg slightly bent, the knee somewhat raised—will plant his left foot, *the toe first*, from thirty to thirty-three inches from the right, and with the right foot will execute what has just been prescribed for the left.

This alternate motion of the legs will take place by throwing the weight of the body on the foot that is planted, and by allowing a natural, oscillatory motion to the arms. The cadence of this step may be increased to more than one hundred and eighty per minute, thus forming *an exercise in running*, the only difference consisting in a greater degree of swiftness. In executing the movements of this Series, *the students should breathe through the nose, keeping the mouth closed.*

IX.

COMBINED EXERCISES.

FIRST SERIES.

First Position.

No. 244.—Thus far, in Calisthenics, we have given one hundred and thirty elementary positions, and two hundred and fifty classes of movements, which require about seven thousand separate motions in their execution. While the rule of Permutation is not strictly applicable in determining the number of *combinations* that may be formed from these elementary positions and movements, it is sufficiently so to prove that they are almost innumerable. After the elementary movements are mastered, combined ones may be executed without previous practice, simply by employing appropriate words of command. The few examples that follow are designed to illustrate the mode of forming these exercises, both by a combination of two or more elementary movements, and by the combined efforts of two students. The ingenious instructor will not find it difficult to form hundreds of new combinations in like manner.

No. 245.—The instructor will command: 1. *Combined Exercises;* 2. *First Series;* 3. *Chest Exercise with Charges;* 4. *First—*Position.

No. 246.—At the fourth command, the student will take the position of Fig. 116.—Execute the movements of this position to the Music on p. 85.

COMBINED EXERCISES. 131

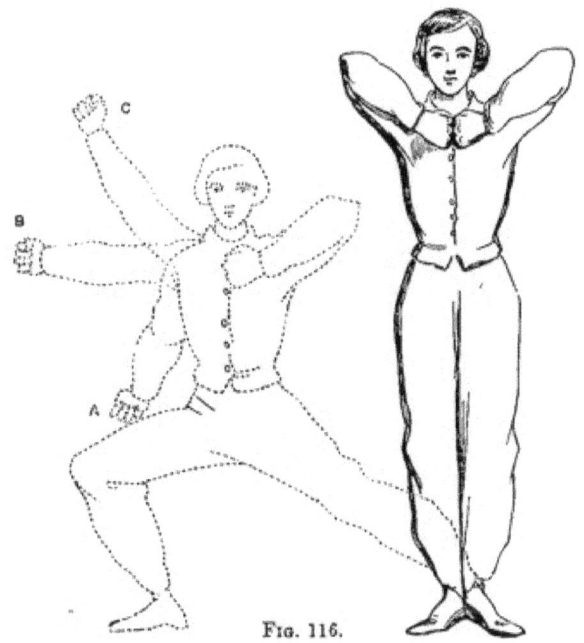

Fig. 116.

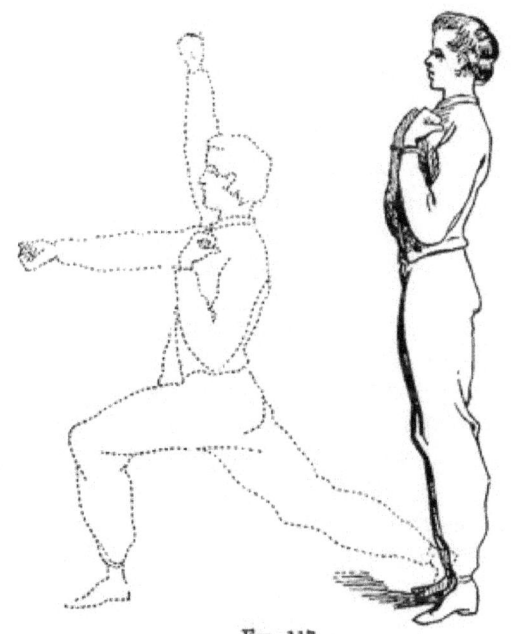

Fig. 117.

No. 247.—*First Movements*—Right. At this command, the student will charge to the right, as represented by the dotted part of Fig. 116, at the same time describing an arc with the right arm to the *right*, inclining down at an angle of 45 degrees, terminating as represented by the dotted arm A, and recover the commencing position four times; then, at the command, Left, four corresponding combined outward motions will be made to the left; and finally, at the command, Alternate, eight of these motions from the commencing position will be made to the right and the left by alternation.

No. 248.—*Second and Third Movements.* These two classes of movements only differ from No. 247 in the directions of the motions from the chest, those of the *second* being directly out to the sides, as shown by the dotted arm B, and those of the *third* sidewise and up, as represented by the dotted arm C.

Second Position.

No. 249.—At the command, *Second*—Position, the student will take the position of Fig. 117, as described in No. 7, p. 34.—Execute the movements of this position to the Music on p. 86.

No. 250.—*First, Second, and Third Movements.* The remaining commands, and the number and order of motions of these three classes of movements, are the same as those of the first position; but the charges and arm motions are made directly front, *the right arm and left leg first*, as represented by the dotted part of Fig. 117, the first class of arm movements being made directly down; the second, directly front; and the third, directly up.

Third Position.

No. 251.—At the command, *Third*—Position, the student will take the position of Fig. 118; see, also, Fig. 15.—Use Part Fourth, p. 104, in connection with the movements of this position.

No. 252.—*First, Second, and Third Movements.* These movements only differ from those of the First Position in having the charges made to the front, inclining to the right and the left at an angle of 45 degrees, see Fig. 118, the first class of arm movements from this position being made front and down, at an angle of 45 degrees; the second, directly front; and the third, front and up, at an angle of 45 degrees; see, also, dotted arms of Fig. 15.

COMBINED EXERCISES. 133

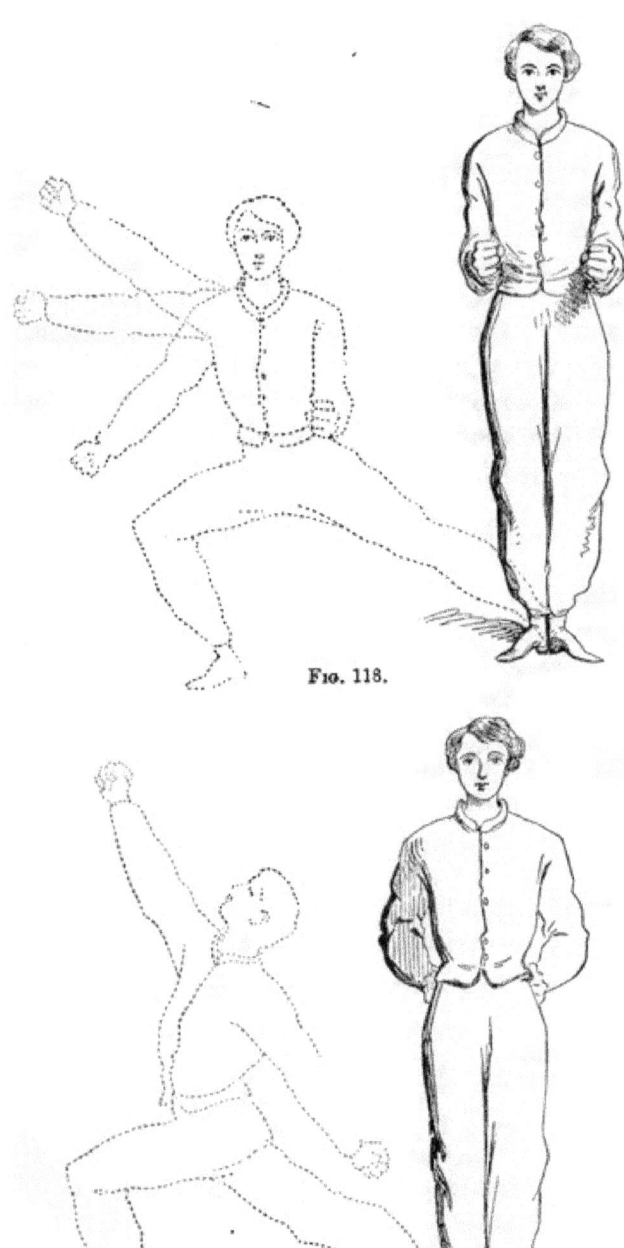

Fig. 118.

Fig. 119.

Fourth Position.

No. 253.—At the command, *Fourth*—POSITION, the student will take the position of Fig. 119; see, also, Fig. 16.—Use Part Fifth, p. 104, with the following class of movements.

No. 254.—*First Movements*—RIGHT. The remaining commands, and the number, order, and direction of the charges of the first and only class of movements from this position, are the same as in No. 233; but in every charge and facing to the right, the right arm is carried front and up at an angle of 45 degrees, and the left arm back and down at the same angle, as represented in the dotted part of Fig. 119. In charging and facing to the left, in like manner the left arm is carried front and up, and the right one back and down.

SECOND SERIES.

First Position.

No. 255.—The instructor will command: 1. *Combined Exercises;* 2. *Second Series;* 3. *Chest Exercise with Marching;* 4. *First*—POSITION.

No. 256.—At the fourth command, the student will take the position of Fig. 120; see, also, No. 2.

No. 257.—*First, Second, and Third Movements.* The first class of movements from the chest is made down and back, at an angle of 45 degrees, as represented by the dotted arm A, Fig. 120; the second, directly out and back horizontally, as shown by the dotted arm B; the third, in the direction of the dotted arm C. The remaining commands, and the num-

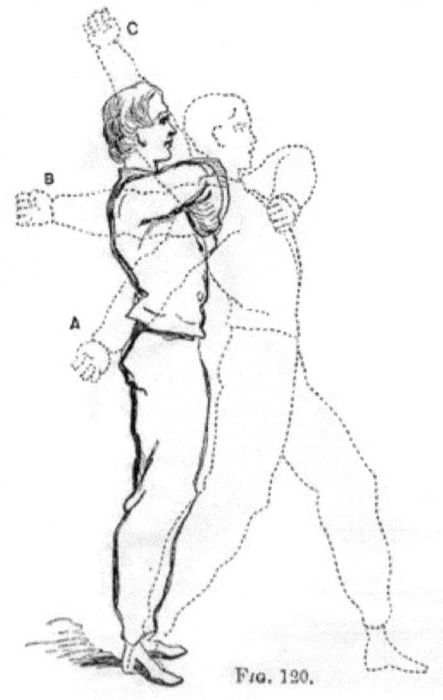

FIG. 120.

ber, order, and kind of motions, are the same as those of Nos. 4, 5, and 6, pp. 32 and 33; but these movements are accompanied with marching, as described in No. 239. *The arm or arms will be out at the greatest distance from the chest every time the left foot is planted, and the commencing position will be regained every time the right foot is planted.*

No. 258.—The Chest Exercise of the second, third, and fourth Positions will be executed as prescribed on pp. 34 and 35, combined with marching, as explained in No. 257. All of the Shoulder Exercise, and most of the movements in Elbow, and Arm and Hand Exercise, may also be executed in combination with marching.

THIRD SERIES.

First Position.

No. 259.—The instructor will command: 1. *Combined Exercises;* 2. *Third Series;* 3. *First*—Position.

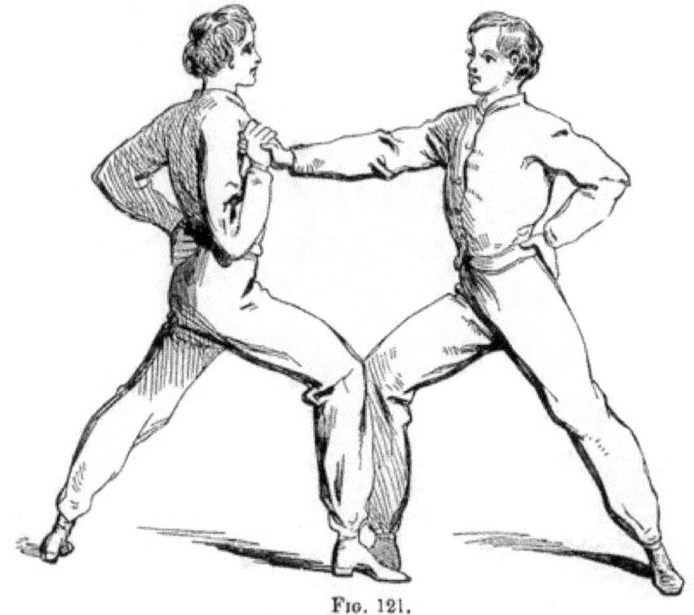

Fig. 121.

No. 260.—*Third Series.* The exercises of this Series are performed by the combined efforts of the students, arranged in couples.

The students will number as prescribed on p. 17, the ones and twos forming partners. Preparatory to this exercise, at the command, *Twos, one pace forward*—March, the twos take a step forward of about thirty inches, and join heels, as in the *military* position; then, at the command, *Twos, About*—Face, the twos will turn to the right on the left heel, describing one-half of a circle, as in No. 193, and face the ones.

No. 261.—At the third command of No. 259, the two ranks will take the position of Fig. 121, the right feet being placed side by side, the right legs bent at the knee, the left legs straight, the feet of each student at right angles to each other, the left hands fixed upon the hip, the right arm of the ones bent as much as possible and held firmly against the right side, and the right hands clasped at arm's-length from the twos, as shown in Fig. 121.

No. 262.—*First Movements.* These movements are executed by first forcing the extended arms of the twos into the position of the ones, as in Fig. 121, and then forcing the extended arms of the ones back to the commencing position sixteen times. In executing these flexions, the arms are held snugly by the sides, the elbows being carried directly back so as to graze the waist, and a slight resistance is offered by the extended arm. The greater the resistance offered, the more effective the movements become.

No. 263.—*Second Movements.* At the command, Change, the position will be taken with the left legs advanced, the right hands fixed upon the hip, and the left hands clasped, the left arm of the twos being bent, and the left arms of the ones extended. These movements, which correspond to those of No. 262, are made with the left arms.

Second Position.

No. 264.—At the command, *Second*—Position, the students will take the position of Fig. 122, in which the right legs are advanced, the feet of each student being at right angles to each other, the arms of the ones are forced back, and the arms of the twos are extended their full length.

No. 265.—*First Movements (Parallel Bars).* The movements of this position correspond to those with parallel vertical bars ||. Each student becomes a pair of *living* parallel bars—a conduit of power—a strength-giving implement, more invigorating than any apparatus of the gymnasium. First, at the command, RIGHT, the right arms of the ones force back the left arms of the twos into a position corresponding to that of the ones, and are immediately forced back into the commencing position four times; then, at the command, LEFT, the left arms of the ones in like manner force back the right arms of the twos and regain the commencing position four times; then, at the command, ALTERNATE, this motion is made, first with the right arms of the ones and then with the left, eight times by alternation; then, at the command, RECIPROCATE, fifteen of these motions are made from the position by reciprocation (eight with the

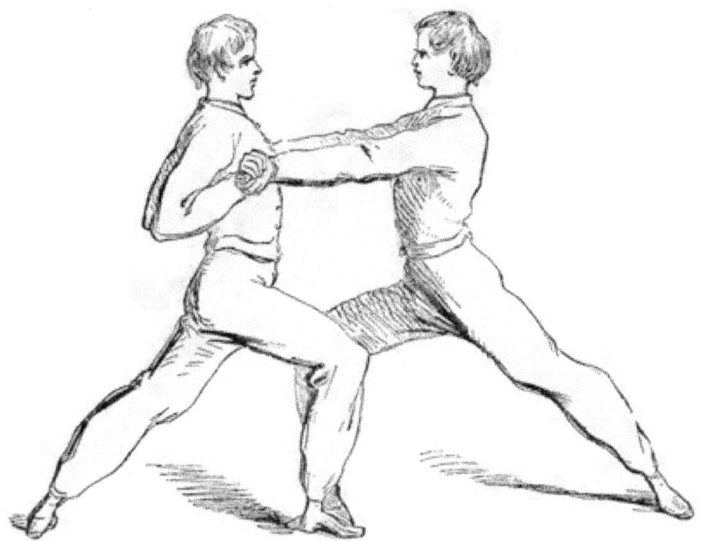

FIG. 122.

right arms of the ones and seven with the left), the left arms of the ones advancing at the same time their right arms are being forced into the commencing position by the twos, and conversely; and finally, at the command, BOTH, the ones force simultaneously both arms of their partners into the position of the ones, and regain the commencing position eight times. In executing these movements, the elbows will be forced directly back, as represented in Fig. 122.

No. 266.—*Second Movements.* At the command, CHANGE, this position will be taken with the left legs advanced, the arms of the twos forced back, and the arms of the ones extended. This class of movements, which corresponds to that of No. 265, is commenced by the twos.

Third Position.

No. 267—At the command, *Third*—POSITION, the students will take the position by turning back to back and standing erect, the ones locking their arms around the arms of the twos, as shown in Fig. 123.

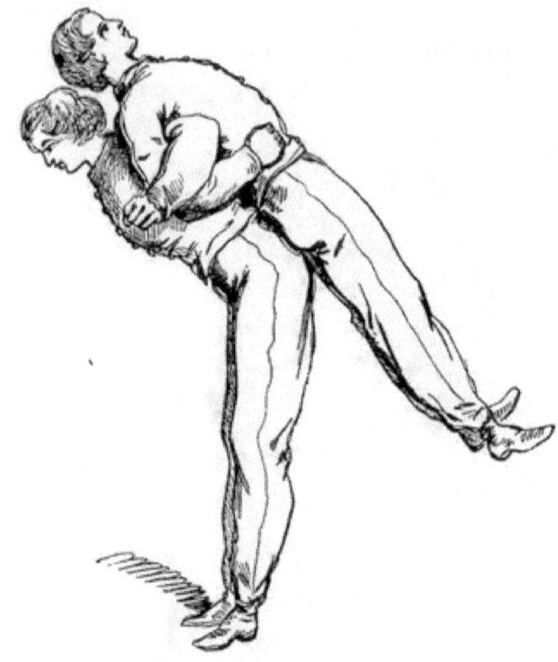

FIG. 123.

No. 268.—*First Movements*—COMMENCE. At this command, the ones lean forward at an angle of 45 degrees, bending only at the hips, lifting the twos, as shown in Fig. 123, and recover the commencing position four times; then, at the command, CHANGE, the twos execute this forward movement, lifting the ones, and recover the commencing position four times; and finally, at the command, ALTERNATE, these forward motions are made eight times from the commencing position by alternation, the ones first lifting the twos and recovering the commencing position.

No. 269.—*Second Movements; Forward*—MARCH. On the word, *Forward*, the ones will lean forward, lifting the twos, as shown in Fig. 123, and, at the last word of the command, they will march forward in this position until they advance thirty-two steps, or the command, CHANGE, is given, when the twos in like manner will lift the ones and march back to their original standings. The two classes of movements of this position bring into play nearly all the muscles and joints of the body, and are specially valuable as exercise for the chest, back, shoulders, and elbows.

FOURTH SERIES.

First Position.

No. 270.—The instructor commands: 1. *Combined Exercises;* 2. *Fourth Series;* 3. *First*—POSITION.

No. 271.—The students will be drawn up in two ranks, standing face to face, at arm's length from each other. At the last command, the twos will take the position of the dotted part of Fig. 124, leaning to the left with the head supported by the right hand, the left hand fixed upon the hip, and the lungs fully inflated.

No. 272.—*First Movements*— BEAT. At this command, the ones will lean forward and beat smartly the right sides of the twos with their palms, up and down from the waist to the armpit, first giving sixteen blows by reciprocation, one hand approaching the side at the same time the other recedes, and then eight double blows, both hands ascending and descending

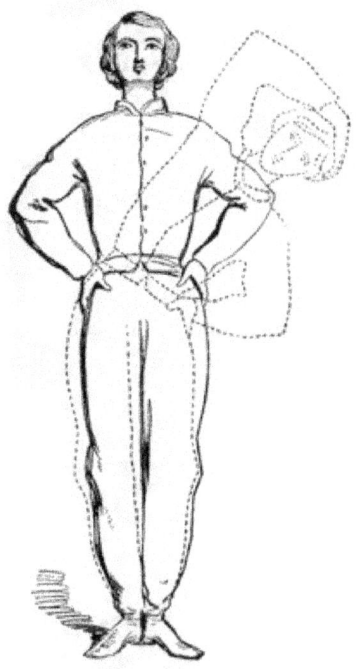

FIG. 124.

simultaneously; when, at the command, CHANGE, the ones instantly take the position, bending sidewise to their right, and the twos in like manner beat the left sides of the ones; then, at the second command, CHANGE, the twos instantly take the position, bending sidewise to their right, and the ones in like manner beat the left sides of the twos; and finally, at the command, CHANGE, the ones instantly take the position, bending sidewise to their left, and the twos in like manner beat the right sides of the ones. These blows are given with great rapidity in connection with Vocal Exercises, pp. 39 to 43, or Music. The best Music for this Series is on pp. 56, 57, and 102.

Second Position.

No. 273.—At the command, *Second*—POSITION, the twos will take the position of the solid part of Fig. 124, in which the hands are fixed upon the hips, the trunk, bent at the hips, inclines back, and the lungs are fully inflated.

No. 274.—*First Movements*—BEAT. The remaining commands, and the number and order of motions, correspond to those of No. 272; but, at the first command, the ones beat the chests of the twos up and down in front; at the second, the twos in like manner beat the chests of the ones in front; at the third command, the twos will face about and incline slightly forward, bending the trunk only at the hips, and the ones will beat the backs of the twos from the waist up and down; and finally, at the last command, the twos will instantly face about into position, and the ones will simultaneously face about, turning their backs toward the twos; when the twos in like manner will beat the backs of the ones. At the command, ATTENTION, the ones will face about, and both ranks will take the *military* position. As this is one of the most useful, as well as most pleasing, of all the Series of exercises in Calisthenics, the instructor will take especial pains to secure the utmost promptitude, precision, and exactness in the execution of the movements.

FIFTH SERIES.

First Position.

No. 275.—The instructor commands: 1. *Combined Exercises;* 2. *Fifth Series (Foot Movements);* 3. *First*—POSITION.

No. 276.—This Series embraces *Movements from the spot done in pairs.* At the third command, the students, formed in two straight lines, will all face in the same direction, each couple standing abreast,

COMBINED EXERCISES.

the line of twos being at the right of the ones; the feet will be placed in *military* position, Fig. 124; the left hands of the ones and the right hands of the twos will be fixed upon the hips, and the left hands of the twos will be sustained by the right hands of the ones, as in Fig. 125.

No. 277.—*First, Second, Third, Fourth,* and *Fifth Movements.* The *first* class of foot movements of this position is the same as No. 238; the *second,* as No. 239; the *third,* as No. 241; the *fourth,* as No. 242; and the *fifth,* as No. 243, the steps being taken simultaneously by the students, arranged in pairs as explained in No. 276.

No. 278.—*Sixth Movements*—FORWARD. At this command, the ones and twos, joining their hands in pairs, simultaneously slide their left feet forward, as seen in Fig. 125, and instantly draw the right feet up to the heel of the left. This movement is repeated until eight slides are taken with the left feet, when the right feet advance and make eight corresponding slides. All of the students thus advance in the same direction, in straight lines; around a room, turning at each corner; or in a circle, until the instructor

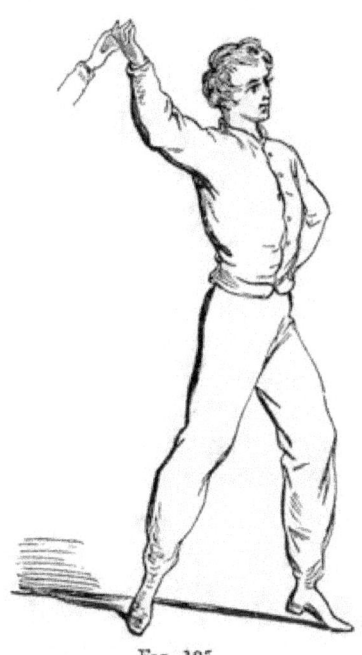

Fig. 125.

commands, *Class*—HALT; or, *About*—FACE. When the last command is given, the students instantly turn round and execute the movements in a contrary direction. The turning is done toward the interior of the room or the center of the circle. This class of movements constitutes what is usually called a *sliding exercise. In all the movements of this Series, the instructor will take especial pains to secure ease, grace, and elasticity, as well as correctness and precision.* Appropriate MUSIC on pp. 57 and 102.

No. 279.—*Seventh Movements*—FORWARD. At this command, the students simultaneously execute a short forward slide, inclining to the left, and a hop with the left foot, and then a corresponding slide and hop with the right foot. These alternate motions continue until the instructor commands, *Class*—HALT; or, *About*—FACE, as in No. 278. The hop that immediately follows each slide, alone varies these movements from the usual motions employed in skating. Music, Part First, p. 102. First, however, employ the second variety of counting, on p. 40.

No. 280.—*Eighth Movements*—FORWARD. In executing this class of movements, the students first slide the left foot forward, inclining toward the left at an angle of 45 degrees, then lift the right foot and place it immediately behind the heel of the left foot, and then hop twice on the left foot; second, the right foot makes a corresponding slide, inclining to the right, the left foot is placed behind the right heel, and then two hops are done with the right foot. These movements are continued until the instructor commands, *Class* —HALT; or, *About*—FACE, as explained in No. 278. Count as in No. 279. Music, Part Second, p. 102.

No. 281.—*Ninth Movements*—FORWARD. This class of movements is formed wholly of hops. The couples advance by first hopping four times on the point of the right foot; then four times on the point of the left foot; and finally, eight times in alternate double hops, the first and second being done on the left foot, the second and third on the right, &c. The students will continue to repeat the movements until otherwise commanded. Music appropriate for this exercise on p. 103.

The instructor will remember, that the students are not to touch their heels to the floor while executing the sixth, seventh, eighth, and ninth classes of movements.

Second Position.

No. 282.—At the command, *Second*—POSITION, the ones and twos will face each other, placing their feet in the *military* position, and standing near together, the ones holding the hands of the twos, with the arms hanging naturally by the sides.

No. 283.—*First Movements*—FORWARD. This class of movements, which corresponds to No. 281, is formed wholly of hops. The couples all advance sidewise in the same direction, the twos within the circle, or nearest the center of the room. They move forward in

COMBINED EXERCISES. 143

the direction of the right arm of the ones, first elevating the advanced legs and arms, as shown in Fig. 126, and executing four simultaneous hops; then the advanced arms are depressed, the arms in the rear elevated at an angle of 45 degrees, and the advanced feet execute four simultaneous hops; and finally, eight simultaneous hops are done, the first and second on the points of the feet in the rear, the third and fourth on the toes of the advanced feet, &c., the advanced arms being elevated whenever the hops are done on the feet in the rear, and lowered every time they are done on the advanced feet. The students continue to advance until the instructor commands, *Class*—HALT; or, *About*—FACE. When the last command is given, the students turn round, as in No. 278, and execute the movements in a contrary direction.

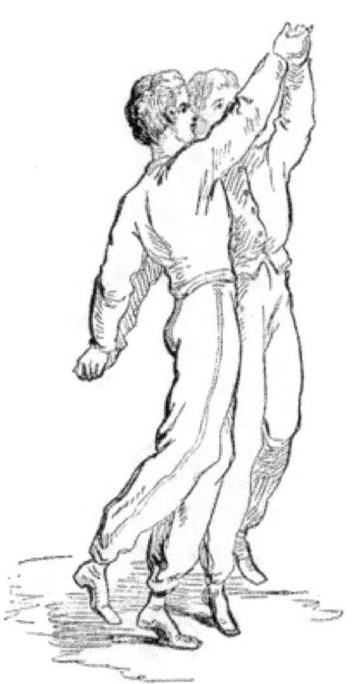

Fig. 126.

No. 284.—*Second Movements* —FORWARD. This class of movements corresponds to the *sliding* exercise of No. 278. With the arms in the position of Fig. 126, the right feet of the ones and the left feet of the twos simultaneously execute eight slides, when the couples instantly turn completely round, lowering the arms that were up, and elevating the ones thus brought to the front, and continue in the same direction, executing simultaneously eight slides with the left feet of the ones and the right feet of the twos, when the commencing position is instantly resumed. The students thus continue until otherwise commanded.

No. 285.—*Third Movements*—FORWARD. The couples, with their arms as in Fig. 126, will simultaneously execute a slide, the ones with the right feet and the twos with the left; then they will immediately lift the feet in the rear, place them just behind the advanced feet, and hop once on the feet thus placed. These three motions will be repeated until the advanced feet execute four slides, when the students will instantly face about, as in No. 284, and execute a like number of corresponding motions in the same direction, the slides being made with the left feet of the ones and the right feet of the twos. These movements will thus continue until otherwise commanded. At first, the students will execute these movements in connection with counting, employing the fourth variety on p. 40. Appropriate Music on p. 105.

No. 286.—*Fourth Movements*—Forward. In the position of Fig. 126, the students will advance, first hopping simultaneously four times with the feet in the rear; and then, lowering the advanced arms and elevating the arms in the rear, they will hop four times with the advanced feet. They will thus continue, changing the feet employed, and the direction of the slant of the arms, on every fourth hop, until sixteen hops are executed. Then the couples will instantly turn so as to bring the twos on the outside of the circle, or nearest the outside of the room, when they will simultaneously execute a slide, the ones with the left feet and the twos with the right, lift the feet in the rear, place them just behind the advanced feet, and hop once on the feet thus placed. This slide, with the two accompanying motions, will be repeated four times; when the couples, instantly recovering their original position with the ones outside, will execute the four slides with the accompanying motions, the ones sliding with the right feet and the twos with the left. This class of movements will be repeated *at pleasure*. The students will first execute the movements in connection with counting, employing the following order, and giving each accented number twice the time of the others: One, two, three, fóur; one, two, three, fóur; one, two, three, fóur; one, two, three, fóur: óne, two, three; óne, two, three; óne, two, three; óne, two, three: óne, two, three; óne, two, three; óne, two, three; óne, two, three. One, two, three, fóur, &c. Music, p. 83.

No. 287.—To secure a greater variety, the students will occasionally execute the first nine classes of movements of this Series in files of four abreast. Nearly all the movements of the Series may be executed in circles, formed by the students taking hold of each other's hands. A pleasing variety is secured by forming the class into three circles, the innermost and outermost circles passing to the right, while the intermediate one passes to the left, and *vice versa*.

WATSON'S
GYMNASTIC APPARATUS.

THIS is the most beautiful, convenient, and effective GYMNASTIC APPARATUS ever devised. It embraces only the few varieties that afford the most and best exercise in the shortest time; that may be used with equal facility under cover, or in the open air; and that may be employed by all persons, either individually or in classes.

It is all made of well-seasoned wood, varnished with three coats of shellac, and well polished. Dumb-bells and Indian Clubs are usually made of maple, beech, or birch; Wands, of white-ash; Hand-rings, of cherry or mahogany. APPARATUS will be manufactured to order, of hickory, locust, rosewood, or lignum-vitæ.

The Wand has eight plane, equal faces, or sides. It is *seven-eighths* of an inch thick for men and women, and *three-fourths* for boys and girls. It extends from the floor to the lobe of the ear. *Price, without metallic balls, 30 cents; with metallic balls, 60 cents.*

There are four sizes of Dumb-bells. No. 1 is intended for men; No. 2, for women and youth; Nos. 3 and 4, for boys and girls. Full descriptions are given on pp. 255 and 256 of this work.—*Price, per pair, of Nos. 1 and 2, 75 cents; of Nos. 3 and 4, 60 cents.*

There are eight sizes of Indian Clubs; four of *long clubs*, and four of *short ones*. Nos. 1 and 2 are intended for men; Nos. 3 and 4, for women and youth. Full descriptions are given on pp. 258 and 259.—*Price of Short Clubs, per pair, $1.25; of Long Clubs, Nos. 1 and 2, $1.75; of Long Clubs, Nos. 3 and 4, $1.50.*

Two sizes of Hand-rings (pp. 260 and 261) afford a sufficient variety. No. 1 is intended for men and women; No. 2, for boys and girls.—*Price, per pair, well polished, 75 cents.*

A liberal deduction from the above prices will be made to Schools and Gymnasiums.

Address

SCHERMERHORN, BANCROFT & CO.,

130 GRAND-STREET, NEW YORK.

WATSON'S
NATIONAL PHONETIC TABLETS.

THESE TABLETS, *eight* in number, each 24 by 30 inches in size, printed in colors and mounted in the best style, may be read at a distance of one hundred feet. They present in the simplest, most convenient and attractive form for class drill, all the excellences of the American phonetic and the English phonic systems, without any of their objectionable features, furnishing abundant and appropriate material for the acquisition of the basis of all good delivery—*a perfect articulation.* This is done as follows:

I. By employing figured vowels and consonants, thus securing just as many distinct characters as there are elementary sounds in the English language, *without the introduction of a single new letter.*

II. By giving a list of all letters and combinations of letters that ever represent these sounds, with the necessary exercises.

III. By furnishing all needful rules, and ample and apposite directions and explanations for instructors.

IV. By an exhaustive, though simple analysis of English words, both as spoken and written.

V. By phonetic reading, embracing many words usually mispronounced, and all the difficult combined sounds of the language, thus securing what may be regarded as a complete vocal gymnasium.

These TABLETS are used in some of the best Academies, Public and Normal Schools, and Gymnasiums of the United States.

Price, mounted on heavy boards in card form, $4.00; *in the best map form,* $6.00.

Address

SCHERMERHORN, BANCROFT & CO.,

130 GRAND-STREET, NEW YORK.

THE HAND-BOOK

OF

CALISTHENICS AND GYMNASTICS.

BY J. MADISON WATSON.

One volume 8vo., tinted paper, with Illustrations from Original Designs, and Music to accompany the Exercises. Price $1.75.

THIS new work is a Drill-Book for Schools and Gymnasiums, and a Hand-Book for individuals and families, containing a complete course of *Exercises both with and without Apparatus.* We submit the following

OPINIONS OF THE PRESS.

THIS volume is divided into three parts, the first, Vocal Gymnastics, devoted to respiration, phonetics, and elocution, including choice poetical selections; the second, to Calisthenics; and the third, to Gymnastics. It is most beautifully illustrated and printed, and as a piece of book-making is highly creditable to the firm whose name is on the title-page. The piano music to accompany the exercises is selected from the favorite composers, and the work is altogether the most complete and elaborate of any yet published on the subject.—*N. Y. Evening Post.*

WE heartily commend this valuable Hand-Book to the notice of our readers—to all who prize physical culture, health, and symmetrical education. We hope it may find its way into our schools and families. Print, paper, and the mechanical execution are really excellent.—*The Continental Monthly.*

A VOLUME both valuable and beautiful. The numerous illustrations are fresh and well drawn, and the proper music accompanies the varied series of exercises. Chapters on Respiration, Orthoëpy, and Expression precede those pertaining to Calisthenics and Gymnastics, and are accompanied with judicious selections for voice culture. In execution, the book surpasses all its predecessors.—*The Independent.*

JUST the book needed for schools, families, and gymnasiums—for the sedentary, and all persons not accustomed to daily manual labor in the open air. The health of the whole community would be promoted if the principles inculcated by this work were more generally known and heeded.—*The New York Observer.*

A VERY useful and particularly handsome book. Its author has herein treated, in a scientific spirit and an agreeable style, a very important branch of education. It teaches the necessity and the best means of educating the human body simultaneously with the human mind. We cordially commend this work to every reader.

It will be found serviceable to all classes of instructors, and to all classes of students.—*The Albion.*

THIS book is very comprehensive in its character, embracing several topics which have never heretofore, so far as we are aware, been included in one treatise. The three divisions are severally manuals on Vocal Culture, Calisthenics, and Gymnastics. In each part, the subject is pursued in a most careful and exact form, and illustrated in a style that leaves nothing to be desired.—*Phila. Sunday-School Times.*

A MOST compendious and reliable hand-book of physical culture. The classes of movements are given not only singly, but in combinations which are as ingenious as they are varied and numerous.—*The Worcester Palladium.*

WE can not speak too highly in praise of the care which has been so elaborately bestowed upon the composition and arrangement of the calisthenic and gymnastic exercises. They are finely worked up, containing many new and elegant combinations. Mr. WATSON has made a happy move in the right direction; and we hope to see a more general interest excited in Calisthenics and Gymnastics inspired by this work.—*N. Y. Teacher.*

AS a hand-book of physical training for individuals, families, schools, and gymnasiums, it has not been equaled by any work which has come to our knowledge.—*Mass. Teacher.*

ONE of the most valuable works of the season. Part first, *Vocal Gymnastics,* is a clear, comprehensive, and eminently practical treatise on respiration, vocal culture, and elocution. The second division, *Calisthenics,* contains a variety of beautiful and useful exercises that are to be executed without apparatus. Part third, *Gymnastics,* embraces the more advanced manual exercises that are to be executed with apparatus. A separate treatise is introduced for each piece of apparatus, affording an inexhaustible variety of carefully elaborated exercises. The book can not be too highly recommended to schools, families, the sedentary, and invalids.—*Home Jour.*

THIS is the most elaborate and satisfactory attempt yet made to apply practically to educational purposes the great truths of physiology, relating to physical culture and training. The work has evidently been prepared by one who is conscious of the requirements of the learner, and has studied the most effectual way of meeting and supplying them. To those in authority, whose influence would be effectual in promoting the circulation of this book, it becomes a positive duty so to do by every means in their power. All who have the physical welfare of the human race at heart, and understand how powerless the intellect is to contend against the burden of a feeble and emaciated frame, are equally interested in its teachings, and answerable, each in his own sphere, however small it be, for the consequences of neglecting them.—*N. Y. Daily Times.*

WATSON'S HAND-BOOK has been adopted by the Board of Education of the City of New York, and it is already used in nearly all of the Public Schools. Single copies sent by mail, on receipt of $1.75 by the Publishers,

SCHERMERHORN, BANCROFT & CO.,
130 Grand Street, New York.
GEO. & C. W. SHERWOOD, CHICAGO.

www.ingramcontent.com/pod-product-compliance
Lightning Source LLC
Chambersburg PA
CBHW031500160426
43195CB00010BB/1048